Improving Sports Performance in Middle and Long-Distance Running

Improving Sports Performance Series

Series Editors

Joanne L. Fallowfield and **David M. Wilkinson**
University College Chichester, Chichester, West Sussex, UK

Series Advisory Panel

Jens Bangsbo
August Krogh Institute
Copenhagen, Denmark

Mark Hargreaves
Deakin University
Burwood, Victoria, Australia

Priscilla M. Clarkson
University of Massachusetts
Amherst, MA, USA

Clyde Williams
Loughborough University
Leicestershire, UK

Athletes from all levels of achievement competing in sport are involved in a continuous quest to optimise performance. The aim of this book series is to present a new synthesis of contemporary knowledge and understanding with respect to the scientific basis of performance. Whilst accepting that there is no one answer, this series aims to provide prescriptive, sports-specific advice as far as is presently possible.

Improving Sports Performance is aimed at three groups of people. First, sports participants aspiring to improve their personal performance through a more complete understanding of the application of science. Second, coaches of such athletes who wish to complement the art of coaching by basing their training programmes upon rational scientific principles. Third, sports science and physical education students with an interest in implementing the theoretical background of their course in an applied sporting context. Thus, this book series sets out to steer a course between the theoretical texts of exercise physiology and biochemistry, and popular coaching texts.

Each book will interrogate the specific physiological mechanisms underpinning performance within each sport, critique current training theories and approaches to preparing for competition, and where appropriate present modified interpretations of these theories in the light of new knowledge and insights. Thus, it is hoped that readers will be in a position to develop a more informed, self-critical, and specifically focused training approach. Whilst it is accepted that this is a very ambitious undertaking from the outset, if at best the series provides an empirical foundation from which to make informed decisions about training and competition preparations, then it will have served its purpose.

Improving Sports Performance in Middle and Long-Distance Running

A Scientific Approach to Race Preparation

Edited by

JOANNE L. FALLOWFIELD AND DAVID M. WILKINSON
School of Sports Studies, University College Chichester, UK

JOHN WILEY & SONS, LTD

Chichester · New York · Weinheim · Brisbane · Singapore · Toronto

Copyright © 1999 by John Wiley & Sons, Ltd,
Baffins Lane, Chichester,
West Sussex PO19 1UD, England

National 01243 779777
International (+44) 1234 779777
e-mail (for orders and customer service enquiries): cs-books@wiley.co.uk
Visit our Home Page on http://www.wiley.co.uk
or http://www.wiley.com

Other Wiley Editorial Offices

John Wiley & Sons, Inc., 605 Third Avenue,
New York, NY 10158-0012, USA

VCH Verlagsgesellschaft mbH, Pappelallee 3,
D-69469 Weinheim, Germany

Jacaranda Wiley Ltd, 33 Park Road, Milton,
Queensland 4064, Australia

John Wiley & Sons (Asia) Pte Ltd, 2 Clementi Loop #02-01,
Jin Xing Distripark, Singapore 129809

John Wiley & Sons (Canada) Ltd, 22 Worchester Road,
Rexdale, Ontario M9W 1L1, Canada

Library of Congress Cataloging-in-Publication Data
Fallowfield, Joanne L.
Improving sports performance in middle and long-distance running : a scientific approach to race preparation/Joanne L. Fallowfield, David M. Wilkinson; (Editors).
p. cm.
Includes bibliographical references and index.
ISBN 0-471-98437-X (alk. paper)
1. Running–Physiological aspects. 2. Running–Training.
I. Wilkinson, David M. II. Title.
RC1220.R8F34 1999
612'.044–dc21
99-28034
CIP

British Library Cataloguing in Publication Data

A catalogue record for this book is available from the British Library

ISBN 0-471-98437-X

Typeset in 10/12pt Times from the author's disks by Keytec Typesetting Ltd., Bridport, Dorset.
Printed and bound in Great Britain by Biddles Ltd, Guildford, Surrey
This book is printed on acid-free paper responsibly manufactured from sustainable forestry, in which at least two trees are planted for each one used for paper production.

For Alex and Joseph
JLF

For Rhona, Matthew and Kate
DMW

Contents

CHAPTER 8: NUTRITION FOR PERFORMANCE

CHAPTER 9: RUNNING AND THE ENVIRONMENT

Biographies of Contributors

Robert B. Child, PhD, is a Post-doctoral Research Fellow at University College Chichester, UK. His research interests lie in exercise-induced muscle damage, specifically focusing upon mechanisms of tissue injury during periods of excessive training stress. He is a keen runner and road cyclist.

Joanne L. Fallowfield, PhD, is a Senior Lecturer in Exercise Physiology at University College Chichester, UK. She was Exercise Physiologist to the England Team for the 1998 Commonwealth Games and is a British Olympic Association and British Association of Sport and Exercise Science accredited Exercise Physiologist.

Alex Twitchen, MA, is a Senior Lecturer in the Sociology of Sport at University College Chichester, UK. His research interests lie in the sociology of sport, consumption and the body. He was a keen club runner, competing in a range of middle and long-distance events.

Peggy Wellington, MPhil, is a freelance Sports Nutritionist. She is a member of the British Olympic Association Nutrition Steering Group, and worked at the 1992 and 1996 Olympic Games, as well as the 1998 Commonwealth Games. In addition, Peggy has worked with a number of elite athletes from a wide range of sports.

David M. Wilkinson, MSc, is a Lecturer in Exercise Physiology at University College Chichester, UK. He is presently researching markers of excessive training stress in long-distance runners. David is a British Olympic Association and British Association of Sport and Exercise Science accredited Exercise Physiologist.

Daniel M. Wood, PhD, is a Lecturer in Exercise Physiology at Cheltenham and Gloucester College of Higher Education, UK. He is currently researching the assessment of maximal oxygen uptake in runners, being a keen long-distance runner himself.

Acknowledgements

The authors would like to acknowledge the assistance of Mr Craig Williams in the preparation of the references and Peggy Wellington for her assistance with Chapter 8.

Key Terms

Every effort has been made to define and explain any technical terms within the context of the relevant chapter. However, there are a number of key terms which specifically relate to the physiology of the middle and long-distance runner, and are repeatedly used throughout the book. For clarity, these terms have also been defined below.

Amino acid: Small nitrogen-containing compounds which link together to form proteins.

ATP: Adenosine triphosphate, the chemical form of energy stored in living cells.

Aerobic metabolism: The processes occurring in cells (muscle fibres) that use oxygen to produce energy (ATP).

Anaerobic: In the absence of oxygen.

Anaerobic capacity: The total AMOUNT of energy that can be obtained from anaerobic metabolism. It is estimated by measuring the maximal accumulated oxygen deficit (MAOD).

Anaerobic metabolism: The processes occurring in cells (muscle fibres) that do not use oxygen to produce energy (ATP).

Anaerobic power: The RATE of energy provision from anaerobic metabolism.

Blood doping: Any means by which an individual's total volume of blood is increased. This is typically achieved by transfusion of red blood cells.

Buffer: A substance that resists change in the acidity or pH, and therefore helps to maintain a constant acid–base (pH) balance.

Buffering capacity: Reflects the capacity available for resisting change in acidity or pH.

Capillarisation: The development (or further development) of a (blood) capillary network to a part of the body. Improved capillarisation of skeletal and heart muscle occurs in response to prolonged endurance training.

Capillary blood: A blood sample obtained from a superficial capillary by way of a finger prick. The ear lobe is another commonly used site for obtaining a capillary blood sample.

Cardiac output: Refers to the volume of blood pumped by the heart per minute, and is measured in litres of blood per minute ($l\,min^{-1}$).

Contractility (of skeletal or heart muscle): The ability of a muscle to shorten forcibly when an adequate stimulus is received.

Economy: A term used to express the oxygen cost required to run at a particular speed. The lower the oxygen cost, the better the running economy.

Effective $\dot{V}O_2$: Represents the oxygen equivalent ($ml\,kg^{-1}$) of the aerobic and anaerobic energy available to sustain race pace running.

Exercise-induced hypoxaemia: The decrease in the oxygen content of arterial blood (hypoxaemia) that occurs in some well-trained endurance athletes during intense exercise.

Glycaemic index: A rating of the increase in blood glucose concentration after the ingestion of a standard amount of dietary carbohydrate. The rating is based on a comparison with the blood glucose response following the ingestion of an equivalent amount of carbohydrate in the form of white bread.

Haemoglobin: The iron-containing pigment in red blood cells that binds oxygen for its transport to tissues, and conversely binds with carbon dioxide in tissue for its transport to the lung.

Hypoxia: A decreased concentration of oxygen.

Interstitial: Relating to the area or space between cells (e.g. between muscle cells).

Lactate threshold: The point during exercise of increasing intensity at which blood lactate concentrations start to increase at a relatively rapid rate.

Lesion: Any structural disruption in a tissue, or loss of function of a body part, which results from some form of damage.

MAOD: An abbreviation representing the maximal accumulated oxygen deficit used to estimate the size of the anaerobic capacity. It is measured in oxygen equivalents and the units are millilitres of oxygen per kilogramme body mass ($ml\,kg^{-1}$).

Metabolism: The sum of all the chemical reactions which take place in the body to sustain life.

Mitochondria (singular mitochondrion): Small structures inside cells that utilise carbohydrates and fats to produce energy aerobically for muscle contraction.

Muscle fibre: An individual muscle cell; the cellular contractile unit which facilitates the application of force through the skeleton, thereby producing or resisting movement.

Myoglobin: A compound similar to haemoglobin, but normally located within muscle tissue. Involved in the transport of oxygen from the cell membrane to the mitochondria.

OBLA: Onset of blood lactate accumulation, or the point at which the blood lactate concentration during exercise of increasing intensity, starts to increase rapidly. Often identified as an exercise intensity (running speed) corresponding to a reference blood lactate concentration of $4.0 \, \text{mmol} \, l^{-1}$.

Osmolality: A measure of the number of particles within a solution; relatively concentrated solutions, which have a high number of particles per kilogramme of fluid, will therefore have a high osmolality.

Oxygenation: The addition of molecules of oxygen; in contrast deoxygenation refers to the removal of molecules of oxygen.

Plasma volume: The portion of the body's total blood volume that is made up of the non-cellular fluid component, plasma.

Staleness: A condition of mental and/or physical fatigue often associated with under performance and/or loss of enthusiasm for training, possibly a consequence of unimaginative, repetitive training sessions or overtraining in extreme conditions.

Stroke volume: Refers to the volume of blood pumped out of the heart each beat and is measured in millilitres (ml).

Total $\dot{V}O_2$ demand: Represents the total energy demand for a particular race, expressed in oxygen equivalent units ($\text{ml} \, \text{kg}^{-1}$).

$\dot{V}O_2$: An abbreviation representing the volume ($\dot{V}$) of oxygen (O_2) taken up by the runner every minute (rate of oxygen uptake). For running it is usually reported in units of millilitres of oxygen per kilogramme body mass per minute ($\text{ml} \, \text{kg}^{-1} \, \text{min}^{-1}$).

$\dot{V}O_2$ demand: The THEORETICAL required rate of oxygen uptake ($\dot{V}O_2$) needed to run at a particular speed. Note that this is a theoretical oxygen demand and does not necessarily mean that the runner can meet this demand, or that this demand is indeed aerobic. For example, running at a $\dot{V}O_2$ demand of $100 \, \text{ml} \, \text{kg}^{-1} \, \text{min}^{-1}$ is well above the $\dot{V}O_{2max}$ for all distance runners and would have to be met by both aerobic and anaerobic energy production.

$\dot{V}O_2$ kinetics: Refers to the rate of increase in $\dot{V}O_2$ at the start of the race.

$\dot{V}O_2$ supply: The ACTUAL rate of oxygen uptake ($\dot{V}O_2$) attained by the runner. It represents the real $\dot{V}O_2$ at a particular point in time and is a measure of the rate of aerobic energy produced by the runner.

$\dot{V}O_{max}$: An abbreviation for maximum oxygen uptake. It represents the maximum rate that a runner can take up oxygen during exhaustive running at sea level.

%$\dot{V}O_2$: The percentage of maximum oxygen uptake. This term can be used to represent the actual $\dot{V}O_2$ supply sustained during a race, or to represent the theoretical $\dot{V}O_2$ demand required during a race, both expressed as a percentage of $\dot{V}O_{2max}$ (%$\dot{V}O_{2max}$). The former is used as a measure of the sustainable %$\dot{V}O_{2max}$ that can be maintained for the duration of a race and represents a purely aerobic component. The latter is used to express the relative exercise intensity of a race, and includes both an aerobic and anaerobic energy contribution. For example, the theoretical relative exercise intensity for an 800 m race may be nearly 130 %$\dot{V}O_{2max}$, but the actual %$\dot{V}O_{2max}$ sustained (or attained) can clearly never exceed 100% $\dot{V}O_{2max}$.

Chapter 1

Introduction

Athletes competing in middle and long-distance running events, from the enthusiastic club runner to the elite professional, are involved in a continuous quest to optimise performance. Hours of dedicated training are undertaken to hone and maximise the body's performance potential in order that a desired outcome is achieved. Yet this process of preparing the body, let alone the mind, for competition is a subject of extensive debate, with many coaches and athletes holding very different beliefs and ideas. These beliefs and ideas are often forged out of traditional and time-honoured practice. Others stem from unquestionably digesting the latest knowledge accumulated by sport and exercise scientists, whilst the practices of successful past athletes are also often used as rigid templates for current athletes to copy.

The aim of this book is not to lay down another training doctrine for athletes and coaches to follow rigidly. Rather the aim is to enable athletes, coaches and students of sports science to acquire a knowledge of contemporary issues concerning the physical preparation necessary for participation in middle and long-distance running events. Nevertheless, as we are all in search of *the answer* that will make us perform better, a framework for prescriptive advice has been presented based upon our current understanding. However, whilst seeking to provide scientifically informed advice as far as possible, it must be remembered that there is no one answer that will satisfy all individual runners. Successful training programmes are based on well-established scientific principles, but adapting these *general* principles to the *specific* needs of the individual is where the boundaries of scientific knowledge merge with the practical experience of the coach. We hope therefore that the chapters in this book will enable the reader to understand more fully and question the physiological mechanisms that underpin middle and long-distance running performance, stimulating reflection on current training strategies, and perhaps even modifying these strategies in the light of new knowledge and insights. In this way a more informed, self-critical and specifically focused training process is likely to lead to a better final product—improved middle and long-distance running performance. From the outset, such an undertaking is extremely ambitious to say the least. However, if at best it gives a runner an empirical foundation from which to make informed decisions about their preparations, it will have served its purpose.

Improving Sports Performance in Middle and Long-Distance Running is therefore aimed at three groups of people. First, middle and long-distance runners who aspire to improve their race times through a more complete understanding of the factors that underpin performance. Second, coaches of such athletes who wish to complement the art of coaching by basing their training programmes upon scientific principles. Third, sports science and physical education students with an interest in implementing the theoretical background of their course in an applied sporting context. Thus, this book sets out to steer a course between the theoretical texts of exercise physiology and biochemistry and popular coaching texts.

Following on from this Introduction, Chapter 2 describes the rate of improvement in middle and long-distance race times over the years, and raises the question as to what extent race times might be further improved. Chapters 3 and 4 investigate the key physiological determinants of middle and long-distance running performance, and present models suggesting how these determinants may interrelate. Chapter 5 examines the nature and extent of adaptability of these determinants with training. Guidance is provided on optimising training approaches in order to address specific training objectives. Chapter 5 also examines variation between well-trained runners to illustrate the limitations imposed by our genetic endowment, as well as discussing ways in which the body may be able to compensate for specific weaknesses by developing other physiological strengths to enable the required performance goal to be achieved. The role of physiological assessment and monitoring in runners is critically examined in Chapter 6, and guidance is given on issues that a runner may wish to consider if they chose to incorporate laboratory or field-based assessment into their training programme.

Training, through necessity, causes tissue damage as part of the process through which tissue is remodelled to more effectively meet the demands of middle and long-distance running. However, inappropriate training will lead to inappropriate and excessive tissue damage which will be disabling rather than enabling to the runner. Some of the causes of tissue damage are discussed in Chapter 7, and strategies are presented that will help a runner to optimise adaptation rather than become another casualty requiring rehabilitation. One such strategy involves ensuring that a runner is provided with an appropriate diet to meet their training and competition needs. Guidance on constructing a runner's diet is presented in Chapter 8, and the *promise* of nutrition in maximising performance is discussed.

Finally, *Improving Sports Performance in Middle and Long-Distance Running* considers the impact of the environment on race performance in Chapter 9. The ways in which the runner must cope with different environmental challenges, and in some circumstances use these challenges to complement their training and race preparation is examined. Advice is presented to aid the runner in modifying their training and preparations to manage in sub-optimal conditions, in order to stay healthy and ultimately (as far as is possible) maintain their race performance.

This book has been written by a group of scientists with a keen commitment to improving sports performance. In its writing, this book could have extended into many volumes—the rows of running texts in the bookstores are testament to this fact. However, from its conception it was always intended to be a digest of the essential information, providing the runner and coach with a theoretical basis from which to interrogate their current training approaches. Whilst accepting that not all runners can be winners, in sharing our knowledge it is hoped that all runners will experience the satisfaction of improving their personal performance levels.

Chapter 2

Improving Running Performance: A Modern Phenomenon

Alex B. Twitchen

INTRODUCTION

The spectacle of middle and long-distance running events being led by a lone athlete competing against the clock in an attempt to break a world record time has become a common feature of some prominent non-championship athletics meetings. Such events attract widespread publicity and reflect a modern cultural fascination with attempts to improve and push back the measurable limits of human performance. The modern Olympic motto of *citius–altius–fortius* (faster–higher–stronger) reflects this fascination, and the pursuit of breaking records fundamentally inherent to this ideology is a feature that according to Guttman (1978) represents a distinguishing characteristic of modern sport. For example, as Guttman explains, the classical civilization of Ancient Greece had no concept of records in the modern sense of the term; a feature highlighted by the fact that the Ancient Greeks had no way of saying '*to set a record*' or to '*break a record*'. The obsession with breaking records is therefore a phenomenon which is specific to the industrialised capitalist societies of the kind which first developed in Western Europe during the eighteenth and nineteenth centuries.

The quantification of running performance since the late nineteenth century into standard units of time, along with the standardisation of distances and types of track, has resulted in modern athletics becoming a sport where improvements in performances are relatively easy to measure and assess. However, the cultural fascination with breaking records, and the improvements in performance this indicates, gives rise to a number of interesting questions and challenges. For example, the extent to which world records might ultimately be improved upon has been a matter of intense speculation, and a number of methods have been employed to predict future performances in middle and long-distance running events. This chapter will examine two approaches, assessing the likelihood of further improvements in performance, and the possible limits to these improvements.

The challenge of pushing back the boundaries of human performance through breaking world records is identical to a more general challenge that all athletes face as they attempt to break their own personal best times. Indeed, athletes, coaches and sports scientists working at all levels, from the competitive recreational runner through to the sport's elite, are engaged in a similar process of improving their personal running performance. That is, their goals are orientated to the challenge of maximising their own potential by developing the physiological mechanisms which underpin running performance. The methods by which this may be achieved are central to the current theories on training, and the aim of this book is to assist all athletes in developing better training regimes through the application of sports science. However, this chapter will also assess the process by which new standards in performance are achieved, such that a clearer view of the cultural conditions underpinning the concept of improving middle and long-distance running performance may be understood.

PREDICTING PERFORMANCE IN MIDDLE AND LONG-DISTANCE RUNNING EVENTS

One approach to predicting future world record times is to plot the pattern of past records, either by race time or average running velocity. This approach is termed regression analysis, and allows a line depicting performance improvement to be determined for each middle and long-distance event. By extending this line into the future, a measure of the possible pattern of further improvement may be obtained.

Figure 2.1 illustrates this approach, where world best times between 1911 and 1998 have been plotted for the men's 10 000 m. The final point of this regression line represents Gebrselassie's world record time of 26:22.75 (average running velocity 22.75 km h^{-1}) set in June 1998. Extending the regression line allows predictions of world record times in 2028 (i.e. 24:53) and 2040 (i.e. 24:15) to be made. In order to achieve these

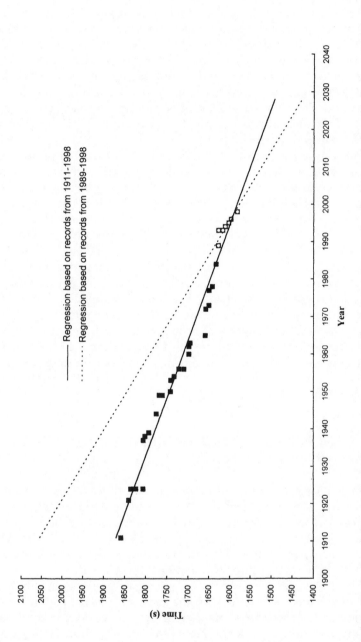

Figure 2.1. Predictions of men's 10 000 m running performance from regression analyses based on records from 1911 to 1998, and records from 1989 to 1998

times, a runner would have to sustain average running velocities of 24.12 and 24.74 km h^{-1} respectively. With respect to the prediction for 2040, this running velocity is some 0.55 m s^{-1} faster than the current world best. In other words, the prediction based on linear regression would suggest that the 10 000 m record breaker of 2040 would complete the event some 800 m—or two laps—ahead of Gebrselassie running at his 1998 world best average race pace.

Regression analysis represents just one possible method of predicting future performances. However, it is a very simplistic method and has a number of limitations which mean that predictions of future performance levels derived from this approach should be treated with caution.

First, any regression analysis needs to be updated continually to account for actual changes in record-breaking performances. This is because predictions of future performances are made based upon a theoretical rate of linear improvement determined from past performance trends. Should actual performances deviate from the predicted trend in any significant way, the regression analysis must be revised in order to accommodate this change in the pattern of performance improvement. Failure to update the regression analysis will result in ever greater errors in a performance prediction.

Second, regression analysis assumes that past performances will serve to influence or limit future performances. That is, the physiological, biomechanical, psychological and environmental factors that influence race performance are subsumed into an historical trend line. As a consequence, regression analysis does not allow an understanding of performance improvement to be developed through a systematic scientific analysis of the determinants of running performance.

A further limitation of regression analysis is that it does not help the athlete, coach or sports scientist to understand why running performances have improved; it merely allows an examination of the rate of improvement to be made. It is therefore not possible from this approach to determine whether an athlete's faster race time has, for example, resulted from a successful training regime, an optimised nutritional strategy, appropriate race preparation or a combination of factors. Thus, we are left to speculate with respect to the reasons underpinning a performance improvement, rather than adopting a systematic review of progress that would facilitate further advancement.

Finally, the ability of a regression line to predict future performance improvements is dependent upon the time frame over which the analysis is performed. It is evident from Figure 2.1 that race times determined from a regression analysis performed on data from 1911 to the present day are distinctly different from those determined by analysing data from 1989 to the present day. Only future actual records will determine which analysis is more accurate and appropriate. Therefore the practical value of regression analysis, based on either running times or average running velocities, to athletes, coaches and sports scientists is questionable.

From the above discussion of the limitations constraining the usefulness of regression analysis, a more sophisticated and potentially more effective method of predicting future performance standards in middle and long-distance running is required. Such an approach is presented by Péronnet and Thibault (1989), who have developed a model that synthesises an awareness of past performance trends in events from the 100 m sprint through to the marathon, with an understanding of the physiological demands underpinning sprint, middle and long-distance running performance. From their analysis, Péronnet and Thibault suggest that improvements in middle and long-distance running performance made during the twentieth century have resulted from general improvements in a runner's maximal oxygen uptake and capacity to produce energy from anaerobic metabolism. The endurance capacity of elite runners has remained seemingly unchanged between 1900 and 1987. The predictions of Péronnet and Thibault for men's events in the years 2000, 2028 and 2040, together with current world records in May 1999 for comparison, are presented in Table 2.1; predictions for women's events in 2000, 2028 and 2033 are presented in Table 2.2.

The analyses of Péronnet and Thibault suggest that considerable improvements in middle and long-distance running performance are still possible. For example, by 2028 Péronnet and Thibault predict a 4.9% improvement in the men's 800 m world record and a 5.6% improvement in the women's 800 m. By 2040 the percentage improvement in the men's event from the current world best is 6.3% and in the women's event by 2033, it is estimated to be 6.0%.

In order to compare two different approaches, the predictions in the tables may be evaluated in relation to the simple regression analysis

Table 2.1. Projection of future world record performances in men's middle and long-distance running events

Event (m)	Year 2000[*]	Year 2028[*]	Year 2040[*]	World record time[†]
800	1:39.88	1:36.18	1.34.71	1:41.11
1500	3:25.45	3:17.45	3:14.27	3:26.00
3000	7:22.54	7:03.91	6:56.87	7:20.67
5000	12:42.72	12:09.39	11:56.19	12:39.36
10 000	26:43.63	25:32.27	25:04.01	26:22.75
42 2000	2:05:23.72	1:59:36.08	1:57:18.47	2:06:05.00

[*] Predictions taken from the data of Péronnet and Thibault (1989).
[†] World record time taken from International Amateur Athletic Federation (IAAF) lists (May 1999).

Table 2.2. Projection of future world record performances in women's middle and long-distance running events

Event (m)	Year 2000[*]	Year 2028[*]	Year 2033[*]	World record time[†]
800	1:51.16	1:46.95	1:46.53	1:53.28
1500	3:47.93	3:38.91	3:38.00	3:50.46
3000	8:11.98	7:50.61	7:48.46	8:06.11
5000	14.19.33	13:41.56	13:37.75	14:28.09
10 000	29:38.41	28:19.04	28:11.04	29:31.78
42 2000	2:18:43.34	2:12:19.55	2:11:40.91	2:20:47.00

[*]Predictions taken from the data of Péronnet and Thibault (1989).
[†]World record time taken from IAAF lists (May 1999).

conducted for the men's 10 000 m event earlier in this chapter. In 2028, the regression analysis forecasts a predicted record of 24:53, whilst Péronnet and Thibault predict a time of 25:32 (i.e. a difference of 39 s). In 2040, the respective predicted race times would be 24:14 and 25:04 (i.e. a difference of 50 s). It is not possible to say prospectively which approach is potentially more *accurate*, though intuitively the more conservative times of Péronnet and Thibault—which incorporate an awareness of the complexity of factors underpinning race performance—would be most appropriate. However, to add a cautionary note, the current world best times for some events in 1999 are better than those predictions made by Péronnet and Thibault in 1989 for the year 2000. Thus, any method of predicting future performances can only ever represent a theoretical 'best estimate' of human potential.

Perhaps of greater interest than speculating on the pattern of performance improvement is to determine the theoretical maximum of middle and long-distance running ability. The predictions of Péronnet and Thibault are based on assumptions of the probable upper limits to human oxygen uptake and anaerobic metabolism capabilities. Tables 2.3 and 2.4 present the predicted ultimate level of performance in men's and women's middle and long-distance running events. For comparison, the world records of May 1999 have been included along with the percentage differences between the predicted ultimate times and current world marks.

Tables 2.3 and 2.4 indicate that, across the range of male and female middle and long-distance running events, the scope of possible improvement up to the theoretically estimated limits of human performance lies between 10 and 14%. However, like regression analysis, the predictions of Péronnet and Thibault are still based on *previous* improvement trends, albeit those that have seemingly taken place in the development of physiological determinants rather than straight performance times or

Table 2.3. Predicted ultimate level of performance in men's middle and long-distance running events

Event (m)	Predicted ultimate level of performance*	Current world record[†]	Percentage difference in performance (%)
800	1:30.96	1:41.11	11
1500	3:04.27	3:26.00	11
3000	6:24.81	7:20.67	13
5000	11:11.61	12:39.36	12
10 000	23:36.89	26:22.75	11
·42 2000	1:48:25.25	2:06:05.00	14

*Predictions taken from the data of Péronnet and Thibault (1989).
[†]World record time taken from IAAF lists (May 1999).

Table 2.4. Predicted ultimate level of performance in women's middle and long-distance running events

Event (m)	Predicted ultimate level of performance*	Current world record[†]	Percentage difference in performance (%)
800	1:42.71	1:53.28	10
1500	3:26.95	3:50.46	11
3000	7:11.42	8:06.11	11
5000	12:33.36	14:28.09	13
10 000	26:19.48	29:31.78	11
42 2000	2:00:33.22	2:20:47.00	14

*Predictions taken from the data of Péronnet and Thibault (1989).

average running velocities. This means that future trends are still based on what we currently know and understand about middle and long-distance running; we cannot predict the *unknown*. It might be that a revolutionary scientific breakthrough may be made, for example in training theory or nutritional supplementation, that significantly enhances human performance potential. As such, future running performances would exceed those currently predicted as the ultimate level of achievement. One example of this would be the pre-marathon nutritional strategies adopted to supercompensate the body's carbohydrate stores developed during the 1960s (Åstrand 1967; refer to Chapter 8 for further details). This scientific breakthrough at the time revolutionised pre-race preparation and greatly improved long-distance running performance. Thus, whilst Péronnet and Thibault predict an ultimate male marathon performance of 1:48:25, future advances in scientific knowledge may mean that this does not necessarily represent the ultimate boundary of performance.

Predicting future record performances in middle and long-distance running is of interest both with respect to the limits of human performance and where current standards of performance are relative to these limits. It therefore provides a frame of reference by which to assess the scope of possible improvements for the future. However, actual improvements in performance are made through a methodical and disciplined approach to training and competition, and without such an approach continuing, it is unlikely that further improvements will be made. Therefore predictions of future running performance assume that a culture which values commitment and hard work, and which rewards success, will remain dominant in modern athletics. But it is also the incorporation of individuals into an ethos of achievement, allied to a scientifically rational approach to training, that has become essential to the process of breaking world records and extending the barriers of human performance.

THE PROCESS OF BREAKING RECORDS

In their study of Kenyan running, Bale and Sang (1996) dismiss the argument that the success of Kenyan athletes is simply due to raw talent combined with an environmental advantage for preparing athletes for middle and long-distance running events. Instead, their analysis highlights the importance of Kenya's incorporation into a westernised global sports culture, Kenya's colonial past and the traditional rivalries within Kenyan society as the important factors that can more adequately explain the success of Kenyan runners.

The status rivalries within Kenyan society have in particular contributed to the Kalenjin (and notably one group of people within this ethnic group, the Nandi) possessing and extolling an ethos of achievement and commitment. This has been essential to the Nandi producing the majority of elite Kenyan runners. The Nandi represent only 1.8% of Kenya's population but in 1988 produced 42.1% of Kenya's elite runners (Bale and Sang 1996). This relatively high degree of success in the Nandi is born out of an ethos of achievement striving, and the use of success in running to demonstrate group status, supplemented by a rational approach to athletic training. Consequently, the phenomenon of Kenyan running is best explained by understanding the development of a cultural way of life that encourages and is conducive to maximising running potential.

Bale and Sang's study reveal a number of insights into the culture of Kenyan running which suggest that simplistic biological explanations for their superior performance standards in middle and long-distance running are unfounded. Thus, it might be argued that improving running performance is about understanding the cultural conditions of social life which create a commitment to maximising the physiological potential of the body. This entails subjecting the body to disciplined and methodical training that is organised around rational training theories and sports science knowledge. Similarly, Gambetta (1993) and Martin (1993) have suggested that the seemingly extraordinary performances of Chinese female athletes might also be understood in relation to their ability to cope, both mentally and physically, with large volumes of intensive training—a capacity which might have much to do with a cultural way of life.

The necessary commitment to disciplined and methodical training is not solely applicable to the challenge of producing world record performances. All competitive athletes, if they are to improve their running performance, need to follow a disciplined training regime that has a rational basis. Consequently, the process of improving performance and breaking records is the same whether the athlete is aspiring to a new world record or looking to break 2 min for 800 m, 16 min for 5000 m, or 3 hours for the marathon. However, we need to consider that the discipline and commitment needed to improve performance, whilst grounded in a cultural way of life, is also related to the cultural value placed on improving performance.

This observation is often overlooked, and the pursuit of constantly aiming to improve performance and break records is assumed to be a timeless characteristic of human societies that can often be explained via *natural* advantages or the use of *unnatural* technologies. But if modern cultures placed little value on the breaking of records, the motivation to conduct the necessary disciplined training to maximise performance would possibly not exist, nor would there be the motivation for scientists to conduct the necessary research to supplement this process. Furthermore, products that promise a quick and relatively easy way of improving performance would not be vigorously marketed or possess any commercial worth. Thus, it is the values of a modern culture that prize an ethos of continuous performance improvement which generates the commitment to training, the incremental accumulation and application of scientific knowledge to human performance, and the desire to go beyond existing limits to performance. In this way, records develop incrementally as athletes and their coaches take up the challenge of surpassing the time which reflects the current limit of human ability.

We can therefore only understand the concept of improving performance in the context of the cultural conditions that generate a desire to improve performance. Equally the success of actually improving performance requires commitment, discipline, hard work and the application of rational training regimes. There are no quick fixes, and though there may be individuals who just possess a natural ability to run quickly over middle and long distances, improving performance at the elite level requires a combination of natural ability with well-organised training and race preparation.

CONCLUSION

This chapter has outlined two approaches by which future performances in middle and long-distance running events might be predicted. The fact that any future performance indicator is only an estimation cannot be over-stressed, but some indicators of potential future performance standards have been given. Whether these standards will be achieved will only become evident in the course of time.

The chapter has also highlighted how the desire to break records, the status given to *record breakers* and the interest in predicting future performance is a reflection of a culture that is fascinated by pushing back measurable performance barriers of all kinds. Yet the process of pushing back performance barriers entails a commitment to hard work and rational training drawing on appropriate scientific knowledge and coaching methods. Thus, the very concept of improving middle and long-distance running performance, and the means by which improvements are achieved are born of a particular set of cultural conditions. These conditions harbour an obsession with breaking records, promoting the values of disciplined commitment, as a necessary prerequisite to this process.

Chapter 3

Physiological Demands of Middle-Distance Running

Daniel M. Wood

INTRODUCTION

This chapter will consider the physiological demands of middle-distance running. Generally, middle-distance track events encompass the 800, 1500 and 3000 m races. However, the 400 m event has also been included for comparative purposes. This event sits uneasily between the sprint events, (i.e. 100, 200 and the rarely run 300 m) and the middle-distance events. From a training perspective, some would view the 400 m as an extended sprint, whilst others would view it as the sprint-end of middle-distance racing. However, with respect to the physiological character-istics of middle-distance running, it will become evident that the attri-butes of a 400 m runner and the attributes of a 3000 m runner represent the extremes of a continuum of determinants of middle-distance running performance. This chapter introduces some of the fundamental physiolo-gical concepts relevant to both middle and long-distance running. These concepts will be examined within the context of middle-distance running, from which a model of performance is developed.

RUNNING SPEED, OXYGEN UPTAKE AND ENERGY PRODUCTION

Running, like any other activity, involves the coordinated contraction of muscles, resulting in the relative movement of parts of the skeleton. The energy required for muscle contraction is provided by the breakdown of the chemical adenosine triphosphate (ATP). The faster the running speed, the faster the rate at which ATP must be broken down and regenerated in the muscle cell (Figure 3.1a). During submaximal running, ATP is regenerated almost entirely from aerobic metabolism (i.e. a series of chemical reactions which require oxygen to break down the fuel from food to produce ATP). Consequently, the relationship between submaximal running speed and the body's rate of oxygen uptake (i.e. the volume of oxygen extracted from inspired air per minute, $\dot{V}O_2$) reflects that between running speed and the rate of ATP breakdown (Figure 3.1b).

The relationship between ATP turnover rate and running speed applies for all running speeds. However, the relationship between $\dot{V}O_2$ and running speed applies only to submaximal speeds. This is because every athlete has an individual maximum rate at which they can use oxygen (i.e. maximum oxygen uptake, or $\dot{V}O_{2max}$). The rate of oxygen uptake cannot exceed $\dot{V}O_{2max}$. As an athlete's running speed increases above that which results in $\dot{V}O_{2max}$, the ATP turnover rate will continue to increase to fuel exercise performance, but $\dot{V}O_2$ is observed to 'level off' or plateau. Thus, to continue to meet the increasing ATP turnover rate, energy must be derived from sources not dependent upon the presence of oxygen (i.e. anaerobic metabolism). The concept of $\dot{V}O_{2max}$ and its relationship with running speed is illustrated in Figure 3.2.

RELATIONSHIP BETWEEN OXYGEN UPTAKE AND RUNNING SPEED

To understand the physiological demands of a particular middle-distance event, it is first necessary to determine the speed that a runner is able to sustain over the distance of the race and to convert this speed into the required rate of oxygen uptake (i.e. $\dot{V}O_2$ demand). This conversion is only possible if the relationship between $\dot{V}O_2$ and track/road running speed is known. From a practical perspective, it is very difficult to measure directly $\dot{V}O_2$ during track running. In contrast, the measurement of $\dot{V}O_2$ whilst an athlete is running on a treadmill is relatively straightforward (Chapter 6), and so the relationship between $\dot{V}O_2$ and treadmill running speed can easily be derived.

The running speed–$\dot{V}O_2$ relationship for treadmill running is generally

---

[1]It is acknowledged that this relationship may not be linear for exercise intensities equivalent to middle-distance race speeds due to the influence of the $\dot{V}O_2$ slow component (Gaesser and Poole 1996). A discussion of the $\dot{V}O_2$ slow component is beyond the scope of this book; however this concept refers to an additional oxygen cost of exercising at moderate to high intensities above that predicted from the running speed-$\dot{V}O_2$ relationship at lower exercise intensities.

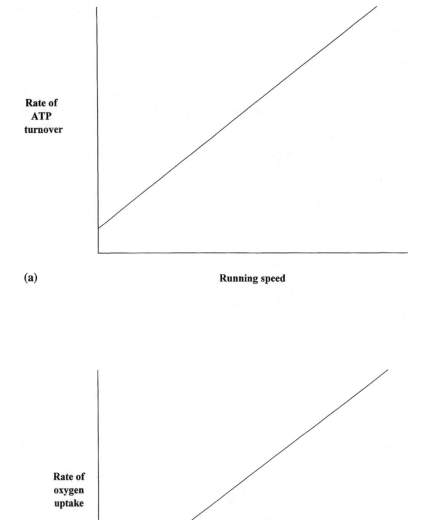

Figure 3.1. (a) Relationship between running speed and the rate of ATP turnover; (b) relationship between running speed and VO_2 during submaximal exercise

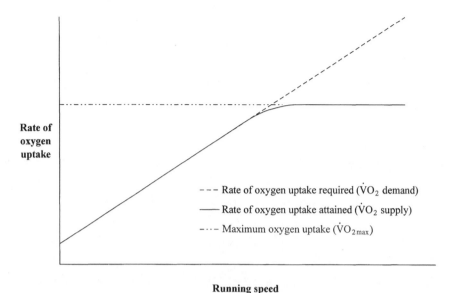

Figure 3.2. Relationship between running speed and $\dot{V}O_2$ for all exercise intensities

considered to be linear[1] throughout the range of human running speeds (Figure 3.3). However, track running differs from treadmill running in that energy is required by the runner to overcome air resistance, something that is not a problem whilst running in one place on a treadmill! The rate of energy production to run on a track at a given speed is therefore the sum of the rate of energy production to run at this speed on a treadmill, and the rate of energy production required to overcome air resistance. This rate of energy production, (usually expressed in terms of an equivalent rate of oxygen uptake), increases as a non-linear (i.e. cubic) function of running speed (di Prampero 1986). This is illustrated in Figure 3.3, where the additional $\dot{V}O_2$ required to overcome air resistance is negligible at slow speeds (i.e. below 13 km h^{-1}) but becomes increasingly significant at faster, race pace speeds. Thus, the running speed–$\dot{V}O_2$ relationship for track running is a combination of a linear (treadmill $\dot{V}O_2$) function and a non-linear (air resistance $\dot{V}O_2$) function. The result is a graph where the line becomes steeper as running speed increases (Figure 3.3).

Figure 3.3 was compiled using data from di Prampero (1986) and would apply to a typical middle-distance runner. The $\dot{V}O_2$ demand to overcome air resistance is proportional to the surface area of a runner, which in turn is relative to a runner's height and body weight. For the purposes of the examples given in this chapter, the typical middle-distance runner is assumed to be 1.75 m tall with a body weight of 60 kg.

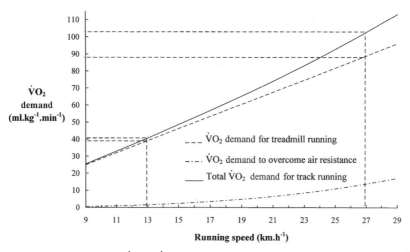

Figure 3.3. Treadmill $\dot{V}O_2$, $\dot{V}O_2$ required to overcome air resistance and total $\dot{V}O_2$ for track running as a function of running speed for a typical middle-distance runner

A runner with a smaller or larger surface area relative to their body mass would require a lower or higher $\dot{V}O_2$ demand respectively to overcome air resistance.

The $\dot{V}O_2$ demand to overcome air resistance when running at the speeds sustained in middle-distance races is considerable, especially for elite runners. For example, when running at $27 \, km \, h^{-1}$ (800 m in 1:47), the $\dot{V}O_2$ demand of a typical middle-distance runner to overcome air resistance is $14 \, ml$ of oxygen per kg body weight per minute ($ml \, kg^{-1} \, min^{-1}$). The total $\dot{V}O_2$ demand to run at this speed would be $103 \, ml \, kg^{-1} \, min^{-1}$ (Figure 3.3). The $\dot{V}O_2$ demand to overcome air resistance therefore represents over 13% of the total $\dot{V}O_2$ demand. Thus, there is a high potential for middle-distance runners to improve their race performance simply by reducing air resistance. This issue will be discussed in greater detail later in this chapter.

AEROBIC AND ANAEROBIC ENERGY PRODUCTION IN MIDDLE-DISTANCE RUNNING

If a typical middle-distance runner had a $\dot{V}O_{2max}$ capable of supplying oxygen to working muscles at a rate of $103 \, ml \, kg^{-1} \, min^{-1}$, they would not be a 'typical' middle-distance runner. The average $\dot{V}O_{2max}$ for this group of athletes is around $75 \, ml \, kg^{-1} \, min^{-1}$ and this will be taken as the $\dot{V}O_{2max}$ for our typical middle-distance runner in this chapter. The difference between the $\dot{V}O_2$ demand ($103\ ml\,kg^{-1}\,min^{-1}$) and the runner's $\dot{V}O_{2max}$ ($75\ ml\,kg^{-1}\,min^{-1}$) represents the anaerobic contribution to energy production, which can similarly be expressed in units of $\dot{V}O_2$ ($103\ ml\,kg^{-1}\,min^{-1} - 75\ ml\,kg^{-1}\,min^{-1} = 28\ ml\,kg^{-1}\,min^{-1}$).

This is illustrated in Figure 3.4 for race pace running during a 400 m and a 1500 m race. It is assumed in this example that the runner reaches their $\dot{V}O_{2max}$ at a running speed of 22 km h^{-1}, and is able to run 1500 m in 3:51 (23.4 km h^{-1}) and 400 m in 0:51 (28.2 km h^{-1}). If energy was only produced aerobically during these events, the $\dot{V}O_2$ demand would be 85.1 ml kg^{-1} min^{-1} (i.e. 113% $\dot{V}O_{2max}$) during the 1500 m race and 108.9 ml kg^{-1} min^{-1} (i.e. 145% $\dot{V}O_{2max}$) during the 400 m race. As the $\dot{V}O_2$ demand is above this runner's $\dot{V}O_{2max}$ for both races, energy will have to be generated anaerobically in these events. Furthermore, as the $\dot{V}O_2$ demand exceeds the $\dot{V}O_{2max}$ by a much greater extent in the 400 m race, the rate of anaerobic energy production will be much higher in this race.

When this analysis is performed for all middle-distance events from 400 to 3000 m, it becomes apparent that in every case the event is completed at a running speed where the $\dot{V}O_2$ demand is greater than the $\dot{V}O_{2max}$. Though notably this difference between the required rate of oxygen demand and the actual rate of oxygen uptake (i.e. $\dot{V}O_2$ supply) decreases as the race distance increases from 400, to 800, to 1500 and eventually to 3000 m. In terms of energy production, this means that

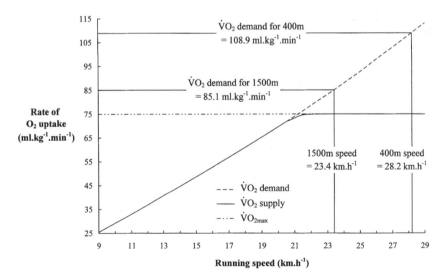

Figure 3.4. $\dot{V}O_2$ demand and $\dot{V}O_2$ supply as a function of running speed for a typical middle-distance runner

some energy must be produced anaerobically in all middle-distance events, but that the rate of anaerobic energy production decreases as the race distance increases.

INTERRELATIONSHIP BETWEEN AEROBIC AND ANAEROBIC ENERGY PRODUCTION IN MIDDLE-DISTANCE RUNNING

The relative aerobic and anaerobic contributions to energy production during middle-distance running are illustrated in Figure 3.5. The total oxygen demand of completing the race is a product of the $\dot{V}O_2$ demand and race duration, whilst the total oxygen supply is a product of the $\dot{V}O_2$ supply and race duration. The total *theoretical* oxygen cost of completing the race is given by the total oxygen demand, whilst the actual oxygen consumed by the runner the race is given by the total oxygen supply.

As discussed previously, the difference between total oxygen demand and total oxygen supply represents the anaerobic contribution to energy production. Thus, the total amount of energy produced during any race

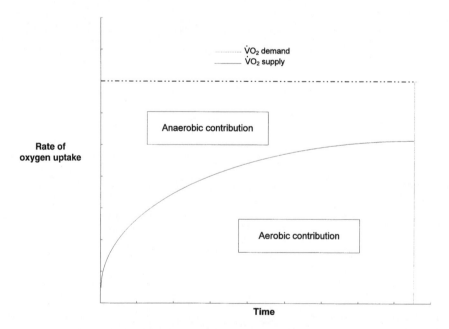

Figure 3.5. Schematic representation of the interrelationship between $\dot{V}O_2$ demand, $\dot{V}O_2$ supply, and the aerobic and anaerobic contributions to energy production

cannot exceed the sum of a runner's anaerobic capacity and the amount of energy that they are able to produce aerobically during the race. Figures 3.6 to 3.9 illustrate the relative aerobic and anaerobic contributions to energy production for our typical middle-distance runner during 400, 800, 1500 and 3000 m races, and are summarised in Table 3.1.

Table 3.1. Aerobic and anaerobic contribution to energy production for 400, 800, 1500 and 3000 m races

Race distance (m) and duration (min:s)	$\dot{V}O_2$ demand (ml kg^{-1} min^{-1})	O_2 uptake required for acceleration (ml kg^{-1})	Total O_2 demand (ml kg^{-1})	Total O_2 supply (ml kg^{-1})	Oxygen equivalent of anaerobic energy production (ml kg^{-1})	% contribution from anaerobic metabolism
400 0:51	108.9	5.9	99	43	56	57
800 1:52	96.3	4.9	185	111	74	40
1500 3:51	85.1	4.0	332	254	78	23
3000 8:15	77.8	3.5	645	570	75	12

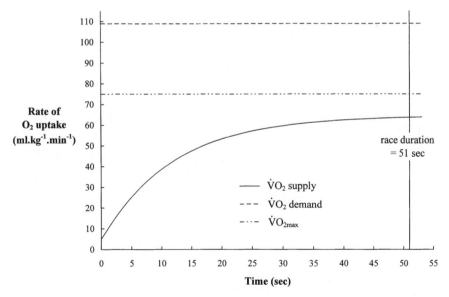

Figure 3.6. Rate of oxygen uptake response for a 400 m race in a typical middle-distance runner

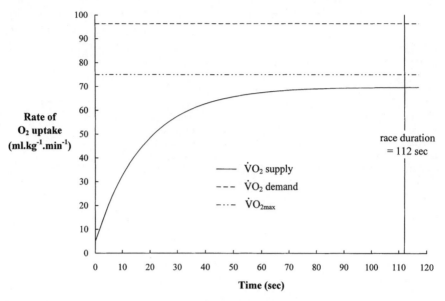

Figure 3.7. Rate of oxygen uptake response for a 800 m race in a typical middle-distance runner

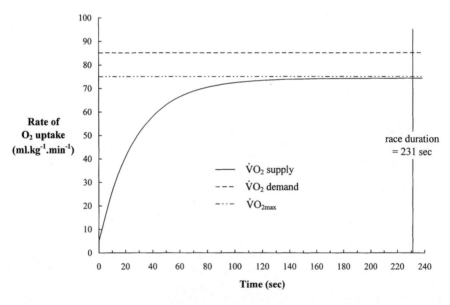

Figure 3.8. Rate of oxygen uptake response for a 1500 m race in a typical middle-distance runner

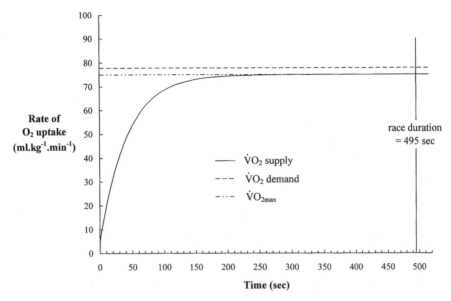

Figure 3.9. Rate of oxygen uptake response for a 3000 m race in a typical middle-distance runner

TECHNICAL BOX 3.1

Calculations Underpinning Figures 3.6–9

In compiling Figures 3.6 to 3.9, the first step was to estimate realistic race times and average running speeds for our typical middle-distance runner for 400 m (0:51, 28.2 km h^{-1}), 800 m (1:52 or 112 s, 25.7 km h^{-1}), 1500 m (3:51 or 231 s, 23.4 km h^{-1}) and 3000 m (8:15 or 495 s, 21.8 km h^{-1}). Each of these average running speeds can be converted into a $\dot{V}O_2$ demand for track running using Figure 3.3. Finally, the total oxygen demand of each event can be calculated by multiplying this $\dot{V}O_2$ demand by the duration of the race. A worked example of this calculation for the 400 m event is presented below.

Example calculation of the relative contributions of aerobic and anaerobic energy production to the total energy demand for the 400 m

- From Figure 3.6, the total oxygen supply attainable for the duration (i.e. 51 s or 0.85 min) of the race is given by the area under the solid ($\dot{V}O_2$ supply) line. This is equivalent to 43 ml of oxygen per kg body weight (ml kg^{-1}).

- The total oxygen demand for the race is given by the area under the dashed ($\dot{V}O_2$ demand) line, and is equivalent to 108.9 ml kg^{-1} min^{-1} × 0.85 min, or 93 ml kg^{-1}. However, the total oxygen demand calculated in this way (i.e. as the product of $\dot{V}O_2$ demand and race duration) only represents the total oxygen demand that would be required to aerobically sustain 28.2 km h^{-1} for 0.85 min and does not include the energy required to accelerate at the start of the race.

- The amount of energy required to accelerate from a stationary start to a given speed is proportional to the final running speed. Furthermore, just as the amount of energy required to sustain 28.2 km h^{-1} for 0.85 min can be expressed as the oxygen uptake that would be required if all this energy was produced aerobically, so the amount of energy required to accelerate to 28.2 km h^{-1} can also be expressed as an equivalent oxygen uptake (i.e. 6 ml kg^{-1} in this case).

- Thus, the combined total oxygen demand equates to (93 + 6) ml kg^{-1} or 99 ml kg^{-1}.

- The oxygen equivalent of the total anaerobic energy production (i.e. the area between the line defining the $\dot{V}O_2$ demand and the line defining the $\dot{V}O_2$ supply on Figure 3.6) equals (99 − 43) ml kg^{-1} or 56 ml kg^{-1}.

- Expressing this as a percentage, anaerobic energy production represents approximately 57% of the total energy demand, with the remaining 43% coming from aerobic energy production.

It is evident that the amount of energy generated aerobically increases with increasing race distance. In contrast, the amount of energy generated anaerobically only increases from 400 to 800 m, with negligible change beyond 800 m (Figure 3.10). Consequently, the percentage of the total energy production derived from anaerobic metabolism decreases, and that derived from aerobic metabolism increases, as the duration of the event increases from 400 to 3000 m (Figure 3.11).

TECHNICAL BOX 3.2

Assumptions Underpinning Figures 3.10 and 3.11

Figures 3.10 and 3.11 are drawn from estimated oxygen uptake data based on *realistic* race performances of our typical middle-distance runner, and assumptions made concerning the relative aerobic and anaerobic contributions to energy production for each event. Presently, there are no means of evaluating the quality of the estimated data and the validity of the assumptions underpinning Figures 3.10 and 3.11 with respect to track-based race performances. This is largely due to the difficulties in collecting oxygen uptake data whilst athletes are running at race pace around a standard 400 m track. However, there are data available from laboratory-based treadmill running studies in which the relative aerobic and anaerobic contribution to energy production has been quantified for supramaximal (i.e. exercise where the $\dot{V}O_2$ demand exceeds $\dot{V}O_{2max}$) exercise bouts of varying duration. Thus:

- The running speed–$\dot{V}O_2$ relationship for submaximal treadmill running can be derived from direct measurements of oxygen uptake over a range of speeds.
- This relationship can be extrapolated to determine the $\dot{V}O_2$ demand for a given supramaximal running speed.
- The $\dot{V}O_2$ supply can be continuously measured throughout a supramaximal treadmill run, and hence the total oxygen supply for this run determined.
- The total oxygen demand can be calculated as the product of the $\dot{V}O_2$ demand (obtained via extrapolation from the running speed–$\dot{V}O_2$ relationship) and the exercise duration.
- The oxygen equivalent of the anaerobic contribution to energy production can be calculated as discussed in Technical Box 3.1.

The only assumption that has to be made in laboratory-based studies is that the $\dot{V}O_2$ demand for a given supramaximal running speed can be predicted from an extrapolation of the submaximal running speed–$\dot{V}O_2$ relationship. Although there is much controversy surrounding the use of this assumption in exercise physiology (refer to Chapter 6) there is presently no satisfactory alternative approach. Nevertheless, accepting this assumption, agreement between the data obtained from laboratory-based studies and those presented in Figures 3.10 and 3.11 would support the appropriateness of the estimated track-based data.

Medbo *et al.* (1988) studied exhaustive treadmill running lasting from 15 seconds up to nine minutes. Anaerobic energy production was observed to increase with increasing exercise duration for exercise bouts lasting less than two minutes, but remained constant for all exercise bouts lasting longer than two minutes (cf. Table 3.1). In a later study, Medbo and Tabata (1989) studied exhaustive cycling exercise lasting between 30 seconds and four minutes. Again it was observed that the amount of energy generated anaerobically increased with increasing exercise duration for exercise bouts lasting less than two minutes, but reached a plateau when the exercise duration exceeded two minutes. Medbo and Tabata (1989) also reported that aerobic energy production increased with exercise duration for exhaustive exercise bouts lasting between 30 seconds and four minutes (cf. Figure 3.10). The relative contribution of aerobic and anaerobic energy metabolism to energy production was examined for exercise bouts lasting 75 seconds and 156 seconds; aerobic metabolism contributed 47% of the total energy production during the shorter exercise bout and 65% during the longer exercise bout. The corresponding percentages estimated from Figure 3.11 are approximately 50% for exercise lasting 75 seconds and approximately 66% for exercise lasting 156 seconds. Thus, again there is good agreement between the data obtained from laboratory-based studies and those presented in Figures 3.10 and 3.11.

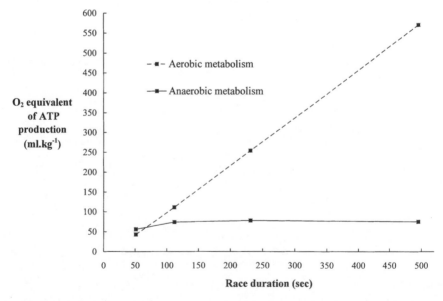

Figure 3.10. Aerobic and anaerobic ATP production as a function of race duration

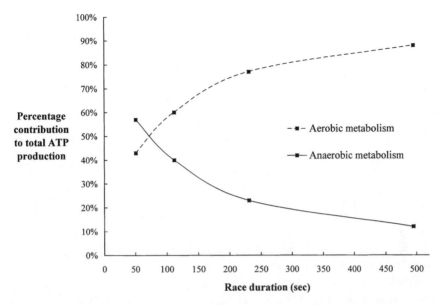

Figure 3.11. Relative contribution of aerobic and anaerobic metabolism to energy production as a function of race duration

There are different limitations to aerobic and anaerobic energy production in middle-distance running. Anaerobic energy production is limited by the total AMOUNT of energy that a runner can generate, which should be constant and equal to their anaerobic capacity. Aerobic energy production is limited by the RATE at which energy can be generated. There is effectively no limit to the total AMOUNT of energy that can be generated aerobically, but the RATE of aerobic energy production is strictly limited by the maximum rate at which a runner can use oxygen (i.e. $\dot{V}O_{2max}$).

If $\dot{V}O_2$ increased to $\dot{V}O_{2max}$ immediately at the start of a middle-distance race, the total amount of energy produced aerobically would only depend on $\dot{V}O_{2max}$ and the duration of the race. However, the rate of oxygen uptake increases gradually at the start of a race, following an exponential pattern. Thus, the total aerobic energy production in a middle-distance race depends not only on $\dot{V}O_{2max}$ and the duration of the race, but also on the rate at which oxygen uptake increases towards $\dot{V}O_{2max}$ at the start of the race ($\dot{V}O_2$ kinetics).

For optimal performance, anaerobic energy production should be spread over the duration of the race, such that the anaerobic capacity is completely exhausted at the end of the race. If a runner does not make a maximal effort, they will not exhaust their anaerobic capacity and their performance would be sub-optimal. Conversely, if a runner starts too quickly, they will exhaust their anaerobic capacity before the end of the race and will 'blow up'. Therefore to achieve an optimal performance, it is necessary to set realistic targets and to adopt a sensible pacing strategy during the race.

TECHNICAL BOX 3.3

Physiological Difference Between the 400 m Event and Other Middle-Distance Events

It seems reasonable to suggest that whilst the duration of an 800 m race would be sufficient to exhaust the anaerobic capacity of even the world's fastest middle-distance runners, this is unlikely to be the case for a 400 m race. This would be consistent with the data presented in Table 3.1, which shows that the oxygen equivalent of the total anaerobic energy production is less in a 400 m ($56 \, ml \, kg^{-1}$) than in an 800 m ($74 \, ml \, kg^{-1}$) a 1500 m ($78 \, ml \, kg^{-1}$) or a 3000 m ($75 \, ml \, kg^{-1}$) race. This highlights why the 400 m race is fundamentally different to the other middle-distance events discussed in this chapter, in that it is the only event in which the anaerobic capacity cannot be exhausted. Thus, training for this event should be focused towards increasing the maximum rate of anaerobic energy production (refer to Chapter 5.)

THE OXYGEN UPTAKE RESPONSE TO MIDDLE-DISTANCE RACES OF VARYING DISTANCE

There are some interesting differences in the $\dot{V}O_2$ response between 800, 1500 and 3000 m races. As the race distance increases, the proportion of the race duration over which oxygen uptake is increasing becomes smaller, decreasing from 90% in an 800 m race (Figure 3.7) through 75% in a 1500 m race (Figure 3.8) to around 50% in a 3000 m race (Figure 3.9). Similarly, the percentage of the maximum oxygen uptake that is reached (i.e. $\% \dot{V}O_{2max}$) during the race increases as the race distance increases (Table 3.2).

The $\dot{V}O_2$ during the race responses shown in Figures 3.7 (800 m) and 3.8 (1500 m) are based on data from a study by Spencer *et al.* (1996), in which well-trained middle-distance runners completed exhaustive treadmill runs at 800 and 1500 m race paces. Oxygen uptake was measured continuously during both runs and $\dot{V}O_{2max}$ was also measured. Both the

Table 3.2. % $\dot{V}O_{2max}$ attained and percentage of total race time taken to reach this final % $\dot{V}O_{2max}$ for 400, 800, 1500 and 3000 m races

Race distance (m)	Race time (min:s)	Estimated $\dot{V}O_2$ demand as % $\dot{V}O_{2max}$	Final $\dot{V}O_2$ attained as % $\dot{V}O_{2max}$	% of time taken to plateau at final % $\dot{V}O_{2max}$
400	0:51.0	145	85	100
800	1:52.0	128	94	90
1500	3:51.0	113	98	75
3000	8:15.0	103	100	50

estimated track data (Figures 3.7 and 3.8) and Spencer's laboratory data show that oxygen uptake reaches a plateau after less time (101 vs 173 s) and at a lower level (94 vs 98% $\dot{V}O_{2max}$) in an 800 m race than in a 1500 m race. In the 3000 m race a runner would reach $\dot{V}O_{2max}$ after 250 seconds (Figure 3.9).

DETERMINANTS OF MIDDLE-DISTANCE RUNNING PERFORMANCE

The total energy required by the muscles for a particular race perform-ance is equal to the sum of the energy required to accelerate to race pace[2] and the energy required to sustain this pace for the duration of the race. Any factor which affects the body's ability to supply energy, or the energy demanded by working muscles, during a race can be considered a determinant of middle-distance running performance.

Determinants of Energy Supply

Anaerobic energy production

The maximum amount of energy that can be generated anaerobically is limited by the size of a runner's anaerobic capacity. Thus, increasing this capacity would improve middle-distance race performance.

---

[2]The initial spurt of energy required to accelerate to race pace is proportional to the square of the speed (i.e. energy for acceleration α race speed^2) and is not affected by any other factors.

Aerobic energy production

The total amount of energy produced aerobically will depend upon $\dot{V}O_2$ kinetics and the final rate of oxygen uptake reached. This final rate of oxygen uptake in the 1500 and 3000 m events would essentially be limited by $\dot{V}O_{2max}$. However, 800 m runners only reach approximately 94% $\dot{V}O_{2max}$ by the end of the race and are therefore limited by the final %$\dot{V}O_{2max}$ that they are able to attain (Table 3.2). In summary, for a particular middle-distance race, the total aerobic energy production will be influenced by $\dot{V}O_2$ kinetics, the %$\dot{V}O_{2max}$ that can be attained in the duration of the race and $\dot{V}O_{2max}$.

Determinants of Energy Demand

In addition to increasing the energy supply, attention should be given to decreasing the energy demanded by the working muscles. Therefore a runner may improve their performance by reducing the energy required to overcome air resistance, or by reducing the energy required to run on a treadmill at race pace.

Overcoming air resistance

The air resistance encountered by a runner when running at a given speed depends on the density of the air and the extent to which a runner is able to 'draft' behind fellow competitors. Air density is influenced by air temperature and air pressure, being highest when the temperature is low and the pressure is high, and lowest when the temperature is high and the pressure is low. Thus, both air temperature and air pressure might be seen as environmental determinants, influencing the energy demand for any middle-distance race performance. With respect to drafting, the air resistance encountered by a runner when running at a given speed is less when running behind other runners. The closer a runner is able to run to the runner in front, the greater the reduction in air resistance. Furthermore, the reduction in air resistance encountered when a small runner runs behind a larger runner will be greater than when both runners are of equal size or a large runner runs behind a smaller runner.

Running speed–$\dot{V}O_2$ relationship for treadmill running—Running economy

As discussed previously, the energy demand of a runner can be expressed as a $\dot{V}O_2$ demand (Figure 3.1). The relationship between the $\dot{V}O_2$ demand and running speed can be derived for submaximal treadmill running speeds, as at these speeds energy is produced almost entirely through aerobic metabolism. Thus, the measured rate of oxygen uptake is assumed to equal the required rate of energy demand. Figure 3.12 illustrates the running speed–$\dot{V}O_2$ relationships for six well-trained runners and the variation between these runners in the rate of oxygen uptake required to run at a speed of 19.3 km h^{-1} (5:00 min mile^{-1} pace).

It is apparent from Figure 3.12 that there is considerable variation between individuals in the oxygen uptake required to run at any given submaximal speed (i.e. running economy). Of the six runners whose data are presented in Figure 3.12, the runner who requires an oxygen uptake of 55.0 ml kg^{-1}min^{-1} to run at 19.3 km h^{-1} would be said to have good economy at this speed. In contrast, the runner who requires an oxygen uptake of 65.9 ml kg^{-1} min^{-1} to run at 19.3 km h^{-1} would be said to have poor economy. Thus, the lower the oxygen consumption to run at a given speed, the better the running economy of a runner at this speed.

Running economy can be assessed for any submaximal speed by measuring the $\dot{V}O_2$ when running at this speed on a treadmill (Chapter 6). However, middle-distance races are completed at speeds for which the $\dot{V}O_2$ demand is greater than $\dot{V}O_{2max}$ (i.e. supramaximal running speeds). The $\dot{V}O_2$ demand cannot be measured at these speeds as it exceeds the

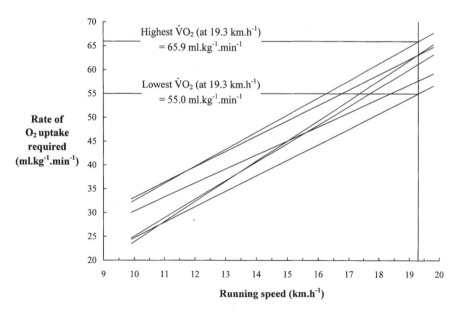

Figure 3.12. Running speed–$\dot{V}O_2$ relationships for six well-trained runners during submaximal treadmill running

maximal attainable value ($\dot{V}O_{2max}$) but it can be predicted by extending the submaximal running speed–$\dot{V}O_2$ relationship (Figure 3.13). The variation between individuals in the $\dot{V}O_2$ demand is illustrated for a speed of 24 km h^{-1} (1500 m in 3:45).

For two runners who differ in running economy to achieve the same performance in a middle-distance race, they must sustain the same average speed throughout the race. The $\dot{V}O_2$ demand to run at this speed will be lowest in the runner with the better running economy. The oxygen cost associated with accelerating to this speed will be the same for both runners, for as discussed previously this only depends on the final speed attained. The total oxygen demand for completing the race (the sum of $\dot{V}O_2$ demand to sustain race pace for the duration of the race and the $\dot{V}O_2$ demand of accelerating to race pace at the start of the race) will be lowest in the runner with the superior economy. Thus, running economy is an important determinant of middle-distance race performance.

A runner who has good economy at submaximal speeds will not necessarily have good economy at supramaximal race pace speeds. This is due to the variation between individuals in the slope of the running speed–$\dot{V}O_2$ relationship (i.e. the rate of increase in $\dot{V}O_2$ with increases in

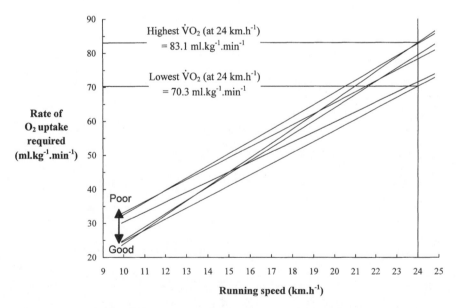

Figure 3.13. Relationship between $\dot{V}O_2$ demand and running speed for six runners during supramaximal treadmill running

running speed) for submaximal treadmill running. This is illustrated in Figure 3.13, where two of the six runners have good economy at submaximal speeds but relatively poor economy at supramaximal speeds, whilst one runner has relatively poor economy at submaximal speeds but good economy at supramaximal speeds. Moreover, the runner who has the best economy at the slowest speed (10 km h^{-1}) has the poorest economy at the highest speed (25 km h^{-1}). Thus, it is not running economy *per se*, but running economy at race speeds that will determine an athlete's middle-distance race performance.

A MODEL OF MIDDLE-DISTANCE PERFORMANCE

Figure 3.14 presents a model of middle-distance running performance in which the determinants of the total capacity to produce energy during a race and the sustainable running speed associated with a given *effective energy*[3] are outlined. The majority of these determinants relate to the physiological characteristics of the runner (i.e. $\dot{V}O_{2max}$, $\dot{V}O_2$ kinetics, anaerobic capacity and running economy), though as has been discussed previously, environmental factors (e.g. air temperature and air pressure) and race strategy (e.g. drafting) must also be taken into consideration. Furthermore, whilst most determinants exert their influence on performance over all race distances, others (those identified by broken lines in Figure 3.14) only exert their influence over some of the race distances within the domain of middle-distance events.

APPLICATION OF THE MODEL OF MIDDLE-DISTANCE RUNNING

The model presented in Figure 3.14 can be used in conjunction with the data presented in Table 3.1 to determine the influence on estimated race time of each determinant of middle-distance running performance. The effects of 10% improvements in $\dot{V}O_{2max}$, $\dot{V}O_2$ kinetics, anaerobic capacity and running economy on performance over 400, 800, 1500 and 3000 m are presented for a typical middle-distance runner in Figure 3.15. These four variables are the only physiological determinants

---

[3]The *effective energy* represents the energy available to sustain race pace running, which represents the total energy demand minus the energy required to accelerate to race pace. The effective energy can be expressed in terms of a rate of oxygen uptake (i.e. effective $\dot{V}O_2$).

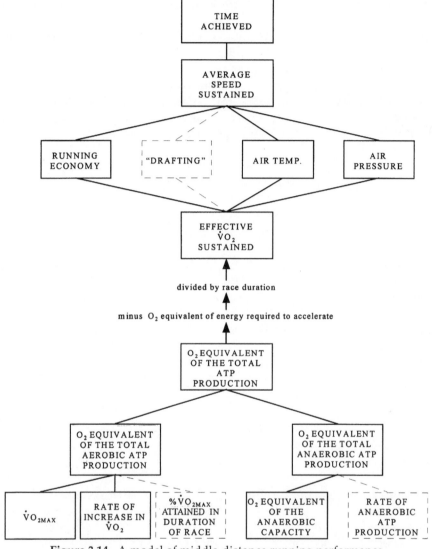

Figure 3.14. A model of middle-distance running performance

which exert an influence on performance across all middle-distance events. It is evident that anaerobic capacity becomes less important and $\dot{V}O_{2max}$ more important, as a determinant of performance, as the race distance increases. Running economy exerts a major influence on performance across all race distances, whilst $\dot{V}O_2$ kinetics is of minor importance.

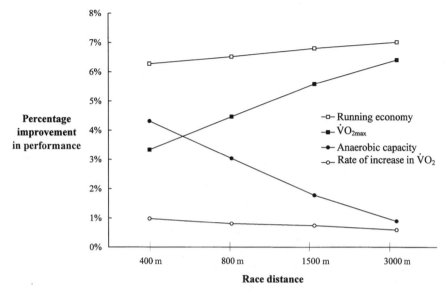

Figure 3.15. Percentage improvements in 400, 800, 1500 and 3000 m performance following 10% improvements in either $\dot{V}O_{2max}$, the rate of increase in $\dot{V}O_2$ (i.e. $\dot{V}O_2$ kinetics), anaerobic capacity or running economy

POTENTIAL IMPACT OF OTHER DETERMINANTS ON MIDDLE-DISTANCE RACE PERFORMANCE

Drafting

When one runner is running behind another, the resulting reduction in air resistance encountered by the following runner varies in relation to the distance between the two runners (i.e. the smaller the distance the greater the reduction in air resistance). However, there is a limit to how small this distance can be, and this minimum distance between runners increases with increasing running speed due to increases in the respective stride lengths of both runners. Kyle (1979) has suggested that a distance of 2 m between runners is realistic at middle-distance race speeds, and with this spacing the following runner will experience a reduction in air resistance of approximately 40%. The $\dot{V}O_2$ demand of a typical middle-distance runner to run alone on a track at 27 km h^{-1} (800 m in 1:47) is 103 ml kg^{-1} min^{-1}, of which 14 ml kg^{-1} min^{-1} is required to overcome air resistance (Figure 3.3). In contrast, if this runner ran 2 m behind another runner, air resistance would be reduced by 40% and the rate of oxygen uptake required to overcome air resistance would decrease by 5.6 ml kg^{-1} min^{-1} (i.e. 40% of 14 ml kg^{-1} min^{-1}). This, in turn, would allow the following drafting runner to sustain a higher speed where the $\dot{V}O_2$ demand would be equivalent to 108.6 ml kg^{-1} min^{-1} (i.e. 103 + 5.6 ml kg^{-1} min^{-1}), or 28.1 km h^{-1}. This increase in sustainable speed from 27.0 to 28.1 km h^{-1} would decrease the 800 m race time from 1:47 to 1:43.

The influence of drafting on race performance is reduced as the race distance increases and the average speed sustained decreases. As the average speed decreases, so does the $\dot{V}O_2$ demand required to overcome air resistance. The race in which drafting might potentially have its greatest impact is therefore the 400 m where the average speed sustained is the fastest of the middle-distance events. However as the 400 m race is run in lanes, it is not possible for competitors to draft fellow athletes. Nevertheless, the impact of drafting on performance in the longer middle-distance events is still significant, so it is important for a runner to try and shelter behind other runners as much as possible in all middle-distance races from 800 to 3000 m.

Air Temperature

As discussed previously, the air resistance encountered by a runner is dependent upon air density, which is in turn dependent upon air temperature. The relationship between air density and temperature is given by:

$$\text{Air density} = \frac{1}{\text{air temperature}}$$

where air temperature is measured on the Kelvin scale and temperature in degrees Kelvin equals temperature in °C + 273.

Seasonal variations in temperature, ranging from 0 °C (i.e. 273 K) to 30 °C (i.e. 303 K), will have commensurate effects upon air density. The air resistance encountered by a runner will be lower in higher temperatures, and though the real effects of changes in air density on race times are relatively small (independent of any seasonal variations in fitness), it is worth bearing in mind that it will always be harder to match summer race performances at colder times of the year.

Air Pressure

Typical air pressures range between 740 and 775 mmHg, a difference of 5%. As air density, and therefore air resistance, is directly proportional to air pressure, the air resistance encountered at race pace may also vary by approximately 5%. For example, a 5% decrease in air resistance could decrease 800 m race time by 0.7 s. In relation to 800 m race times, the impact of air pressure on performance is relatively small, though the practical significance is that it would be harder to achieve a personal best on a high-pressure day in comparison with a low-pressure day.

Effect of Wind

The wind encountered by a runner during track running will also exert an influence across all middle-distance events. The work that must be done by a runner to maintain race pace will increase when running into the wind and decrease when running with the wind. This work done can be translated into changes in the $\dot{V}O_2$ demand and unfortunately these two opposing effects are not equal. Davies (1980) measured a runner's rate of oxygen uptake during treadmill running at a fixed speed with either a head wind or a following tail wind. Not surprisingly, oxygen uptake increased when running into the wind, but this increase was found to be approximately twice as large as the reduction in oxygen uptake observed when runners ran with the wind. The practical implication of these findings, especially with respect to track running on a windy day, is that a runner will not be able to accelerate sufficiently with the wind to compensate for the time lost when running against the wind. Consequently, it will always be harder to achieve a particular race performance on a windy day in comparison to a calm day.

KEY POINTS

- The relationship between running speed and the energy requirements of contracting muscle is reflected in the relationship between running speed and the rate of oxgyen uptake (i.e. $\dot{V}O_2$).
- Energy to fuel middle-distance running is derived from both anaerobic and aerobic metabolism.
- The total energy (oxygen) demand of race pace running is the sum of the energy required to run at a set pace on a treadmill and the energy required to overcome air resistance.
- The relative contributions of anaerobic and aerobic energy metabolism are dependent upon the race duration, which in turn is inversely related to running speed (race pace).
- The total amount of energy generated aerobically during middle-distance running depends upon both $\dot{V}O_{2max}$ and $\dot{V}O_2$ kinetics.
- During optimal middle-distance race performances, the runner's pacing strategy should be such that their anaerobic capacity will be exhausted as the race ends.

- The typical middle-distance runner will reach 94% $\dot{V}O_{2max}$ in the 800 m, 98% $\dot{V}O_{2max}$ in the 1500 m, and 100% $\dot{V}O_{2max}$ approximately half-way through the 3000 m event.
- The amount of energy required to produce a given race performance must equal to the available effective energy, which in turn will determine the average race pace sustained.
- The air resistance acting against a middle-distance runner is proportional to their running speed—faster runners encounter greater air resistance.
- Air resistance is also influenced by local environmental conditions, being reduced when ambient temperature increases and air pressure decreases. A runner can reduce their air resistance by drafting behind fellow runners.

Chapter 4

Physiological Demands of Long-Distance Running

Daniel M. Wood

INTRODUCTION

This chapter considers the physiological demands of long-distance running, encompassing events from 5000 m to the marathon (42.2 km). There are many events that will fit into this long-distance classification: on the track 5000 and 10 000 m races are common; whilst on the road, races have been held over 5 km, 5 miles (8 km), 10 km, 15 km (particularly in the USA), 10 miles (16.1 km), 21.1 km (half-marathon), 20 miles (32.2 km) and 42.2 km (marathon). However, aside from the 5000 and 10 000 m track races, the only distance races for which world championships are currently held are the half-marathon and the marathon. Therefore, the examples given in this chapter will focus primarily on performance over these four world championship distances.

This chapter will not generally distinguish between track races and flat road races as it is assumed that the determinants of performance for 5000 and 10 000 m track races and for flat 5 or 10 km road races are the same. This assumption will be true if the physiological demands of road and track racing are similar. No data are presently available addressing this issue, but it would seem that these are appropriate working assumptions to make. The effect of hill climbing and hill descending on performance in a road race will be considered as a separate issue later in the chapter. Distances will generally be given in kilometres (km) and data presented for 5 and 10 km races are applicable to both track and flat road races.

DEFINING A TYPICAL LONG-DISTANCE RUNNER

As in Chapter 3, this chapter applies concepts relating to long-distance running performance to a 'typical' long-distance runner. However, the spread of distance events make it more appropriate to describe two typical long-distance runners: the middle–long distance runner (M–LD) and the distance runner (DR). The data presented in this chapter were derived from published data (Londeree 1986, Pollock 1977a,b) on two groups of elite long-distance runners. One group comprised M–LD runners whose best distances lay between 1500 and 10 000 m and who were described as 'primarily 3- to 6-milers' (Pollock 1977a). However, as these races have since been replaced by 5 km (3.1 miles) and 10 km (6.2 miles) races, the M–LD group are likely to be mostly 5–10 km runners. The DR group comprised specialist marathon runners.

The data defining the typical long-distance runner represent the combined average data of the two groups. The average performance times for this typical runner are 13:27 for 3 miles, 28:12 for 6 miles and 2:21:30 for the marathon (Pollock 1977a), which are representative of a typical long-distance runner's race times. The average speed required to achieve each of these race times was calculated and the relationship between average speed sustained and race distance was derived (Figure 4.1).

From this relationship it can be calculated that the typical long-distance runner competing at 5 km, 10 km and half-marathon sustains average

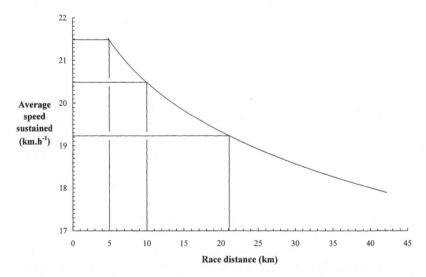

Figure 4.1. Determination of the average speed sustained by a typical long-distance runner for race distances of 5, 10 and 21.1 km

speeds of 21.5, 20.5 and 19.2 $km\,h^{-1}$ respectively. These speeds correspond to times of 13:57, 29:16 and 1:05:56 for the three distances. Extrapolating this relationship to a 42.2 km (marathon) race yields a race time of 2:21:30. The mean $\dot{V}O_{2max}$ of the M–LD and DR groups were 78.8 and 74.1 $ml\,kg^{-1}\,min^{-1}$ respectively (Pollock 1977b). Thus, the $\dot{V}O_{2max}$ for the typical distance runner referred to in this chapter is 76.5 $ml\,kg^{-1}\,min^{-1}$, the averaged value from 78.8 and 74.1 $ml\,kg^{-1}\,min^{-1}$.

RELATIONSHIP BETWEEN OXYGEN UPTAKE AND RUNNING SPEED

Data from Londeree (1986) were used to determine the $\dot{V}O_2$ required by a typical long-distance runner to sustain treadmill running at 3 miles, 6 miles and the marathon race speeds. The $\dot{V}O_2$ required by this runner to overcome air resistance during track/road running was also determined using di Prampero's (1986) formula. For this calculation it was assumed that the height and weight of a typical long-distance runner were 1.76 m and 62.6 kg respectively[1]. These two relationships were then combined to derive a running speed–$\dot{V}O_2$ relationship for track/road running (Figure 4.2).

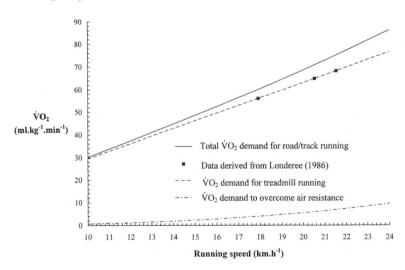

Figure 4.2. The relationship between $\dot{V}O_2$ demand (for road/track running) and running speed for a typical long-distance runner

---

[1]These data for height and weight were obtained from the mean of the M–LD and DR groups (Londeree 1986, Pollock 1977a,b).

AEROBIC AND ANAEROBIC ENERGY PRODUCTION DURING LONG-DISTANCE RUNNING

From Chapter 3 you will recall that $\dot{V}O_2$ demand is the theoretical rate of oxygen uptake that would be required to run at race pace. The $\dot{V}O_2$ supply represents the actual $\dot{V}O_2$ measured during running at this speed. The difference between the estimated $\dot{V}O_2$ demand and the measured $\dot{V}O_2$ supply represents the rate at which energy must be produced anaerobically to sustain the race pace. Figure 4.3 represents the relationship between $\dot{V}O_2$ demand, $\dot{V}O_2$ supply and running speed. The determination of $\dot{V}O_2$ demand and $\dot{V}O_2$ supply is illustrated for race pace running during a 5 km event and a marathon for a typical long-distance runner (i.e. $\dot{V}O_{2max}$ 76.5 ml kg^{-1} min^{-1}, 5 km race time 13:57 and marathon race time 2:21:30).

Similar to Figure 3.4 in Chapter 3, the line representing $\dot{V}O_2$ supply is indistinguishable from that representing the $\dot{V}O_2$ demand for all speeds up to approximately 19 km h^{-1}. As running speed increases above 19 km h^{-1}, these two lines diverge and the difference between $\dot{V}O_2$ supply and $\dot{V}O_2$ demand increases. Thus, the rate of anaerobic energy production for a typical long-distance runner is negligible for all speeds below 19 km h^{-1}, but progressively increases as running speed increases above 19 km h^{-1}. As the average speed sustained for this runner during a

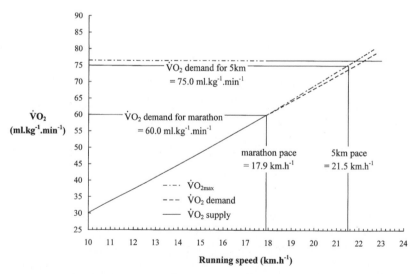

Figure 4.3. $\dot{V}O_2$ demand and $\dot{V}O_2$ supply as a function of running speed for a typical long-distance runner

marathon is $17.9\,\mathrm{km\,h^{-1}}$ and for a half-marathon is $19.2\,\mathrm{km\,h^{-1}}$ (Figure 4.3), it would be reasonable to conclude that the anaerobic contribution to energy production is negligible in both these events. However, this conclusion does not take into consideration the necessary anaerobic contribution at the start of a race, when the $\dot{V}O_2$ is increasing from resting levels. Consistent with observations reported in Chapter 3, the importance of anaerobic energy production during a race increases as race distance decreases.

THE OXYGEN UPTAKE RESPONSE TO LONG-DISTANCE RACES OF VARYING DISTANCE

Figures 4.4–4.7 present the estimated oxygen uptake response for a typical long-distance runner during 5 km, 10 km, half-marathon and marathon events. The $\dot{V}O_2$ demand to run at race pace and the final rate of oxygen uptake attained (i.e. $\dot{V}O_2$ supply) was determined for each event from the running speed–$\dot{V}O_2$ relationship presented in Figure 4.3.

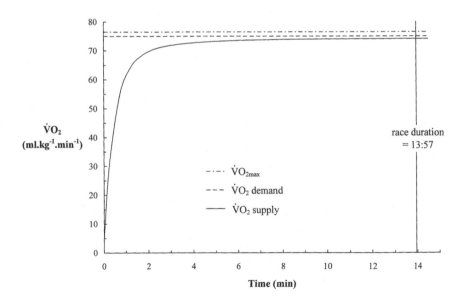

Figure 4.4. Rate of oxygen uptake response for a 5 km race in a typical long-distance runner

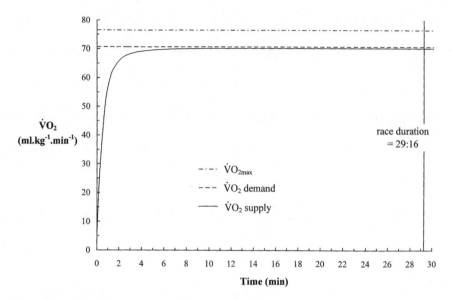

Figure 4.5. Rate of oxygen uptake response for a 10 km race in a typical long-distance runner

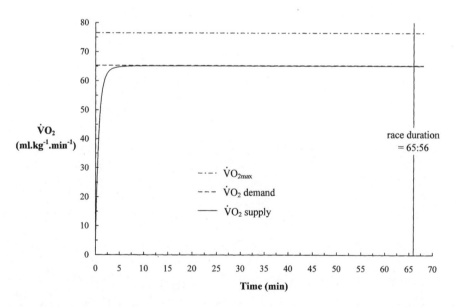

Figure 4.6. Rate of oxygen uptake response for a half-marathon race in a typical long-distance runner

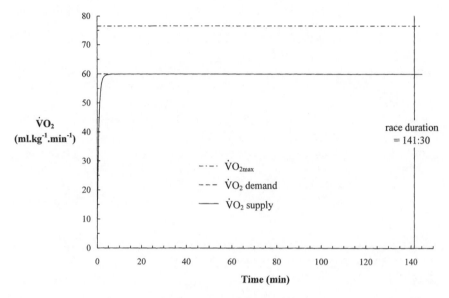

Figure 4.7. Rate of oxygen uptake response for a marathon race in a typical long-distance runner

TECHNICAL BOX 4.1

Assumptions Underpinning Figures 4.4–4.7

Figure 4.4 was drawn from data collected from five runners who completed an exhaustive treadmill run at a speed that required a rate of oxygen uptake equivalent to 97% $\dot{V}O_{2max}$. Similarly, Figure 4.6 was drawn from data collected from 20 runners who completed a 20 min treadmill run at a speed that required a rate of oxygen uptake equivalent to 86% $\dot{V}O_{2max}$. The rate of oxygen uptake required by a typical long-distance runner ($\dot{V}O_{2max}$ of 76.5 ml kg^{-1} min^{-1}) to run at 5 km race pace (21.5 km h^{-1}) is 75.0 ml kg^{-1} min^{-1} (i.e. 98% $\dot{V}O_{2max}$), and to run at half-marathon race pace (19.2 km h^{-1}) is 65.3 ml kg^{-1} min^{-1} (i.e. 85% $\dot{V}O_{2max}$) (Figure 4.3). Thus, the exercise intensity of the treadmill run from which Figure 4.4 was drawn is very similar to that sustained during a 5 km race (i.e. 97 vs 98% $\dot{V}O_{2max}$) and the intensity of the treadmill run from which Figure 4.6 was drawn is very similar to that sustained during a half-marathon race (i.e. 86 vs 85% $\dot{V}O_{2max}$).

The rate of oxygen uptake was measured throughout each of the treadmill runs, from which an average $\dot{V}O_2$ response was determined. During the exhaustive treadmill run, at a speed equivalent to 5 km race pace, the rate of oxygen uptake increased throughout the run and plateaued after approximately 12 min. In contrast, the rate of oxygen uptake during the 20 min treadmill run, at a speed equivalent to half-marathon race pace, plateaued after approximately 8 min. In drawing Figures 4.5 and 4.7 it was assumed that, if the rate of oxygen uptake plateaued after 12 min during a 5 km race and after 8 min during a half-marathon race, the rate of oxygen uptake would plateau after approximately 10 min during a 10 km race and after approximately 6 min during a marathon.

COMPARISON OF THE OXYGEN UPTAKE RESPONSE TO MIDDLE-DISTANCE AND LONG-DISTANCE RUNNING

There are several differences between the $\dot{V}O_2$ responses during long-distance running events (5 to 42.2 km; Figures 4.4–4.7) and middle-distance running events (800 to 3000 m; Figures 3.7–3.9). Through examining these differences it is possible to distinguish between the physiological determinants of middle and long-distance running respectively and hence provide greater understanding for structuring appropriate training programmes.

Proportion of the Race over which the Rate of Oxygen Uptake is Increasing

From Figures 4.4–4.7, it is apparent that the rate of oxygen uptake is essentially constant for the majority of any long-distance race. Furthermore, the longer the race, the smaller the proportion of the total race duration in which $\dot{V}O_2$ is increasing. You will recall that this was not the case during middle-distance events; $\dot{V}O_2$ only plateaued during the latter stages of the 800 m race (Figure 3.7) and even during a 3000 m race $\dot{V}O_2$ did not plateau until half-way through the event (Figure 3.9). Thus, the rate at which $\dot{V}O_2$ increases at the start of a race is more important in determining performance in a middle-distance event than it is in a long-distance event. With respect to long-distance running, this rate would have the greatest impact on race time in a 5 km event, though this would still be relatively small.

The Difference between the Final Rate of Oxygen Uptake Attained and the Required Rate of Oxygen Uptake

The rate of oxygen uptake required to run at race pace during any middle-distance event is greater than a runner's $\dot{V}O_{2max}$. Therefore, there is a significant contribution from anaerobic energy metabolism during these events. In contrast, as the $\dot{V}O_2$ demand during long-distance events is less than a runner's $\dot{V}O_{2max}$, it seems intuitive to suggest all the energy is derived from aerobic energy metabolism. However, $\dot{V}O_2$ supply is only equal to $\dot{V}O_2$ demand during marathon running. Thus, as race distance decreases the difference between $\dot{V}O_2$ demand and $\dot{V}O_2$ supply increases. This would indicate an increasing anaerobic contribution to a runner's total energy requirements as race distance decreases. However, in comparison with middle-distance events, the anaerobic contribution is relatively small.

INTERRELATIONSHIP BETWEEN AEROBIC AND ANAEROBIC ENERGY PRODUCTION DURING LONG-DISTANCE RUNNING

From Figures 4.4–4.7 it is possible to determine the relative aerobic and anaerobic contributions to energy production during long-distance running events (Table 4.1). The calculations from which the data in Table 4.1 were derived are described in Technical Box 4.2.

Table 4.1. Aerobic and anaerobic contribution to energy production for 5, 10, 21.1 and 42.2 km races

Race distance (km) and duration (min:s)	$\dot{V}O_2$ demand (ml kg^{-1} min^{-1})	O_2 uptake required for acceleration (ml kg^{-1})	Total O_2 demand (ml kg^{-1})	Total O_2 supply (ml kg^{-1})	O_2 equivalent of anaerobic energy production (ml kg^{-1})	% contribution from anaerobic metabolism
5 13:57	75.0	3.4	1049	987	62	5.9
10 29:16	70.7	3.1	2072	2010	62	3.0
21.1 65:56	65.3	2.7	4308	4255	53	1.2
42.2 141:30	60.0	2.4	8492	8452	40	0.5

TECHNICAL BOX 4.2

The Principal behind the Calculations Underpinning Figures 4.4–4.7

The actual calculations are the same as appeared in Chapter 3 for determining the relative aerobic and anaerobic contributions to energy production during middle-distance events. However, to illustrate these calculations within the context of a long-distance event, data from Figure 4.4 will be used in determining the contributions of aerobic and anaerobic metabolism to energy production of a typical long-distance runner during a 5 km race.

In completing a 5 km race in 13:57 (i.e. 13.95 min), a typical long-distance runner will sustain an average speed 21.5 km h^{-1}. The rate of oxygen uptake required to sustain this race pace (i.e. $\dot{V}O_2$ demand), assuming that all the energy was produced aerobically, is 75 ml kg^{-1} min^{-1} (Figure 4.3) and the total oxygen demand is 75.0 ml kg^{-1} min^{-1} × 13.95 min or 1046.3 ml kg^{-1}. However, this would not include the additional energy required to accelerate from a stationary start to a race pace of 21.5 km h^{-1} (i.e. 3.4 ml kg^{-1}) and so the complete oxygen demand for this 5 km race is (1046.3 + 3.4) ml kg^{-1} or 1049.7 ml kg^{-1}. The $\dot{V}O_2$ supply during the race would be 987.3 ml kg^{-1}; this deficit between the $\dot{V}O_2$ demand and the $\dot{V}O_2$ supply is met through anaerobic energy production. Thus, the oxygen equivalent of the total amount of energy produced anaerobically during the 5 km race would equal (1049.7 − 987.3) ml kg^{-1} or 62.4 ml kg^{-1}. The oxygen equivalent of the total (aerobic and anaerobic) energy production is given by the complete oxygen demand (i.e. 1049.7 ml kg^{-1}). Therefore for a typical long-distance runner, anaerobic energy production (i.e. 62.4 ml kg^{-1}) represents 5.9% of the total energy production during a 5 km race. Similar calculations determining the aerobic and anaerobic contributions to the total energy requirement can be performed for race distances of 10, 21.1 and 42.2 km.

Anaerobic energy production represents a very small proportion of the total energy production during long-distance races (Table 4.1). Furthermore, both the percentage contribution of anaerobic energy production to the total energy production and the absolute amount of energy generated anaerobically decrease as race distance increases beyond 10 km. The only events in which the anaerobic capacity of a typical long-distance runner may become exhausted would be the 5 km and the 10 km races. This runner would only use approximately 85% of their anaerobic capacity in a half-marathon race and 65% in a marathon race. From Figures 4.6 and 4.7, it is evident that the majority of this anaerobic energy production would occur in the first few minutes of the race. As discussed previously $\dot{V}O_2$ supply equals $\dot{V}O_2$ demand after 8 min in a half-marathon race and after 6 min in a marathon race. Therefore, anaerobic metabolism will only make a significant contribution to the total energy demand during these initial periods.

As anaerobic metabolism represents a relatively small proportion of the total energy requirement during long-distance running, anaerobic power (i.e. the maximum rate at which energy can be generated anaerobically) and anaerobic capacity (i.e. the total amount of energy that can be generated anaerobically) do not appear to be important physiological determinants of long-distance running performance. The impact of any increase in the anaerobic capabilities of a runner would be greatest for the 5 km race. However, this would only have a meaningful effect on performance if there was a substantial increase. It is unlikely that training alone would result in such an increase, but differences in anaerobic capacity between athletes can be large. These differences might explain some of the variation between individuals in the relative exercise intensity (theoretical % $\dot{V}O_{2max}$ sustained during 5 and 10 km races.

RELATIVE EXERCISE INTENSITY SUSTAINED DURING LONG-DISTANCE RUNNING

From the running speed–$\dot{V}O_2$ relationship illustrated in Figure 4.3, the rate of oxygen uptake required by a typical long-distance runner to sustain race pace for 5 km would be $75.0 \, ml \, kg^{-1} \, min^{-1}$ (i.e. 98.0% $\dot{V}O_{2max}$) and for the marathon would be $60.0 \, ml \, kg^{-1} \, min^{-1}$ (i.e. 78.4% $\dot{V}O_{2max}$). Although not shown in Figure 4.3, this relationship can also be used to calculate the rate of oxygen uptake and hence the relative exercise intensity, required to sustain race pace during a 10 km race (i.e. 70.7 ml $kg^{-1} \, min^{-1}$; 92.4% $\dot{V}O_{2max}$) and the half-marathon (i.e. $65.3 \, ml \, kg^{-1} \, min^{-1}$; 85.4% $\dot{V}O_{2max}$).

Figure 4.3 was derived by combining the data of Londeree (1986) for middle–long distance runners (5/10 km) and specialist marathon runners. However, if we now consider the running speed–$\dot{V}O_2$ relationship for each of these groups of long-distance runners separately, the relative exercise intensities sustained by each group for the range of long-distance events can be determined. These are illustrated in Figure 4.8, in which a comparison is made with the typical long-distance runner described in this chapter.

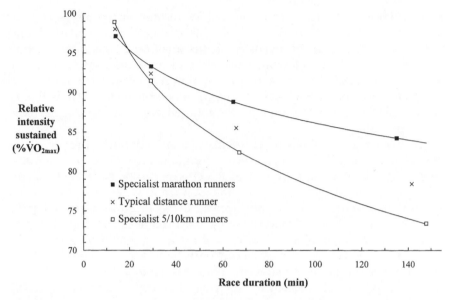

Figure 4.8. Relationship between relative exercise intensity sustained and race duration for middle–long distance runners and specialist marathon runners

The relative exercise intensity sustained by specialist marathon runners declines very little in comparison to that sustained by middle–long distance runners as race duration increases (Figure 4.8). The relative exercise intensity sustained by both groups is similar for events lasting less than approximately 30 min (i.e. 5–10 km). For a race duration of 140 min, the relative exercise intensity sustained by marathon runners (84% $\dot{V}O_{2max}$) is higher than that sustained by middle–long distance runners (74% $\dot{V}O_{2max}$). The relative exercise intensity a runner is able to sustain for a race duration of 140 min is almost entirely dependent upon the actual % $\dot{V}O_{2max}$ sustained over this race time; this means that the influences of anaerobic energy production and the rate at which oxygen uptake increases are negligible. Thus, it would appear that marathon runners are able to sustain a much higher rate of oxygen uptake (relative to $\dot{V}O_{2max}$) for longer duration events in comparison with middle–long distance runners.

TECHNICAL BOX 4.3

Factors Influencing % $\dot{V}O_{2max}$ Sustained during Long-Distance Running

To understand why two runners might sustain quite different rates of oxygen uptake despite having a similar $\dot{V}O_{2max}$, it is necessary to consider the factors that would normally limit $\dot{V}O_{2max}$ and the way in which these factors differ from those determining the $\%\dot{V}O_{2max}$ sustained for a given event.

Exercise physiologists have debated for many years whether $\dot{V}O_{2max}$ is limited by *central* factors relating to the delivery of oxygen to the working muscles, or *peripheral* factors relating to the ability of these muscles to use oxygen at a high rate. Aside from postural muscles of the trunk and counter movements of the arms, it is the leg muscles that are most active during middle and long-distance running. So the question is: which is greater, the maximum rate at which the leg muscles can use oxygen or the maximum rate at which the cardiovascular system can supply these muscles with oxygen? The present consensus, though not universally accepted (Noakes 1991, Powers, Martin and Dodd 1993), is that the rate at which muscles can use oxygen is far greater than the rate at which the cardiovascular system can supply these muscles with oxygen (Poole and Richardson 1997). It would therefore seem reasonable to conclude that $\dot{V}O_{2max}$ during running is primarily limited by central factors determining the maximum rate at which oxygen can be delivered to leg muscles. Of the central factors, the most important appears to be the maximum pumping ability of the heart (i.e. maximum cardiac output). It is important to note that the ability of the leg muscles to use oxygen could differ markedly between two runners with the same maximum cardiac output, and hence a similar $\dot{V}O_{2max}$.

The ability of a muscle to use oxygen at a high rate is referred to as its oxidative capacity. This capacity is influenced by the relative proportions of the different muscle fibres that make up the muscle (Ivy *et al.* 1980). Muscle is not a homogenous tissue; it is made up of different fibre types which are functionally divided into three categories. Type-I fibres are relatively fatigue resistant, having a high oxidative capacity, but a relatively slow rate of contraction (i.e. slow twitch fibres). Type-II fibres have a lower oxidative capacity and are not as fatigue resistant, but have a relatively faster speed of contraction (i.e. fast twitch fibres). Type-II fibres are further differentiated into type-IIa and type-IIb, where the former have a higher oxidative capacity and therefore greater resistance to fatigue. Type-I fibres have a greater number of mitochondria, the organelle within the fibre responsible for the aerobic production of energy. They also have a relatively high concentration of aerobic enzymes, proteins which act as biological catalysts to accelerate chemical reactions, in this case in the aerobic production of energy.

Veteran 10 km runners have been shown to sustain a higher $\%\dot{V}O_{2max}$ than performance-matched younger runners (Allen *et al.* 1985). One explanation is that the concentrations of several key aerobic enzymes are higher in the muscles of the older runners in comparison with the younger runners (Coggan *et al.* 1990). Furthermore, Coyle *et al.* (1991) observed in a group of elite endurance cyclists that those who were able to sustain the highest $\%\dot{V}O_{2max}$ for an 'all out' effort over one hour also had the highest proportion of slow twitch (type-I) fibres, the highest capillary density and the highest concentrations of aerobic enzymes in their thigh muscles.

Thus, it appears that the oxidative capacity of the active muscles is an important determinant of the $\%\dot{V}O_{2max}$ that a long-distance runner is able to sustain for events of 10 km and longer. However, oxidative capacity is not an important determinant of the maximal rate of oxygen uptake ($\dot{V}O_{2max}$) that can be reached during treadmill running. It is possible that a marathon runner could have a lower $\dot{V}O_{2max}$ than a middle–long distance runner despite having leg muscles with a higher oxidative capacity. This would also explain why marathon specialists are able to sustain a higher relative exercise intensity for race distances of 10 km and longer (Figure 4.8). Moreover, just as the proportion of slow twitch fibres, the mitochondrial density, the capillary density and the concentrations of aerobic enzymes in the active muscle are all likely determinants of the $\%\dot{V}O_{2max}$ sustained by an endurance athlete (Coyle *et al.* 1988), they are also determinants of the $\%\dot{V}O_{2max}$ at which lactate starts to accumulate (Ivy *et al.* 1980) in blood (i.e. the $\%\dot{V}O_{2max}$ at which the lactate threshold occurs or onset of blood lactate accumulation, OBLA) (Sjödin, Jacobs and Svedenhag 1982).

An increase in blood lactate concentration would indicate a significant increase in anaerobic energy production. Thus, the lactate threshold would be expected to occur at a higher $\%\dot{V}O_{2max}$ in a marathon runner than in a middle–long distance runner. This is because the marathon runner would have superior aerobic capabilities relative to their $\dot{V}O_{2max}$. However, differences in the oxidative capacity of the leg muscles between a marathon runner and a middle–long distance runner would only explain why the former is able to sustain a higher relative exercise intensity for race distances of 10 km and longer. These differences would not explain why middle–long distance runners are able to sustain a higher relative exercise intensity than marathon runners for a shorter event such as a 5 km race (Figure 4.8). One explanation for this observation might be that the anaerobic capacity of middle–long distance runners is greater than that of specialist marathon runners (Figure 4.9).

RELATIVE EXERCISE INTENSITY SUSTAINED AS A DETERMINANT OF LONG-DISTANCE RUNNING PERFORMANCE

The relative exercise intensity that can be sustained during a long-distance event is an important determinant of long-distance running performance. This is because $\dot{V}O_{2max}$ and the $\%\dot{V}O_{2max}$ sustained interact to determine the effective rate of oxygen uptake (i.e. effective $\dot{V}O_2$) that can be sustained for the duration of a race. It is the effective $\dot{V}O_2$ which, in turn, will determine a runner's race performance. This is illustrated for a typical long-distance runner competing in a 5 km race and a 42.2 km race in Figure 4.10.

The variation between long-distance runners with respect to their sustainable percentage is illustrated in Figure 4.8. The impact that this

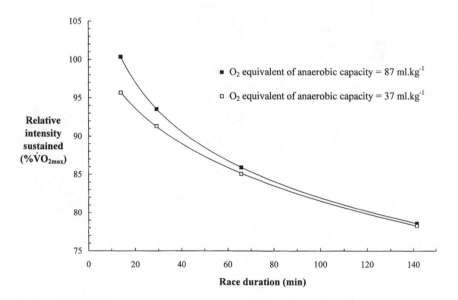

Figure 4.9. Effect of anaerobic capacity on the relationship between relative intensity sustained and race duration

variation will have on long-distance race performance is presented in Table 4.2. The race time associated with each relative exercise intensity was determined for a typical long-distance runner by calculating the effective $\dot{V}O_2$ that would be sustained for a given relative exercise intensity (assuming no change in $\dot{V}O_{2max}$) and then calculating the running speed sustained associated with this effective $\dot{V}O_2$ sustained (Figure 4.10).

The potential for long-distance running performance to be influenced by the relative exercise intensity sustained increases as the race distance increases. This might be one explanation why $\dot{V}O_{2max}$ tends to be lower

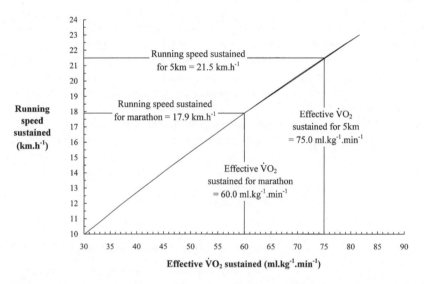

Figure 4.10. Relationship between effective $\dot{V}O_2$ sustained and running speed sustained for a typical long-distance runner

Table 4.2. Effect of relative exercise intensity sustained (expressed as % $\dot{V}O_{2max}$) on the time achieved for race distances of 5, 10, 21.1 and 42.2 km

Race distance (km)	% $\dot{V}O_{2max}$ sustained by M–LD distance runners, i.e. 5–10 km	% $\dot{V}O_{2max}$ sustained by marathon runners	Theoretical time achieved by M–LD distance runners (min:s)	Theoretical time achieved by marathon runners (min:s)
5	98.7	97.2	13:52	14:03
10	91.4	93.3	29:32	29:02
21.1	82.7	88.7	67:38	63:51
42.2	73.9	83.9	148:30	133:41

in marathon specialists than in runners who specialise in the shorter long-distance events (Pollock 1977b, Svedenhag and Sjödin 1984). Runners possessing a relatively low $\dot{V}O_{2max}$ are able to compensate by sustaining a high relative exercise intensity for the duration of a race. A good example of this would be the famous marathon runner Derek Clayton, who held the world record of 2:08:33 throughout the 1970s despite having a $\dot{V}O_{2max}$ of *only* 69.7 ml kg^{-1} min^{-1} (Costill *et al.* 1971b). The two reasons why Clayton was able to perform so well at the marathon distance were: first, he was able to sustain an exceptionally high relative exercise intensity (91% $\dot{V}O_{2max}$) for the duration of the marathon and second, he had good running economy.

RUNNING ECONOMY AS A DETERMINANT OF LONG-DISTANCE RUNNING PERFORMANCE

As discussed in Chapter 3, there is considerable variation between individuals with respect to the $\dot{V}O_2$ required to run at a given speed (i.e. running economy). Figure 4.11 illustrates the running speed–$\dot{V}O_2$ rela-

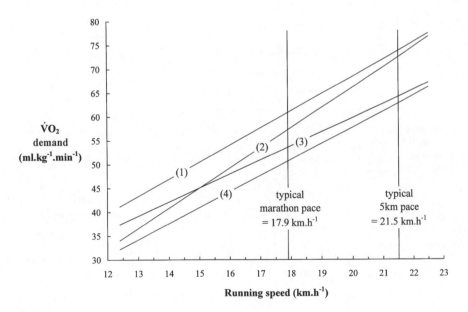

Figure 4.11. Relationship between $\dot{V}O_2$ demand and (treadmill) running speed for four runners

tionships for four of the six runners included in Figure 3.11. The data from the remaining two runners have been omitted for clarity.

There is considerable variation between athletes with respect to both the $\dot{V}O_2$ required to run at a given speed and the slope (i.e. gradient) of the line defining the relationship between the $\dot{V}O_2$ and running speed (Figure 4.11). The slope of the running speed–$\dot{V}O_2$ line is the *same* for runners (1) and (4). This means that the $\dot{V}O_2$ required by runner (1) will *always* be approximately 10 ml kg^{-1} min^{-1} higher than that required by runner (4), regardless of the running speed at which these runners are compared. In contrast, the slope of the running speed–$\dot{V}O_2$ line is much *steeper* for runner (2) than it is for runner (3). As a consequence, the difference between the $\dot{V}O_2$ required by runner (2) and that required by runner (3) is 3–4 ml kg^{-1} min^{-1} at marathon race pace (17.9 km h^{-1}) but is 7–8 ml kg^{-1} min^{-1} at 5 km race pace (21.5 km h^{-1}).

Figure 4.12 emphasises the importance of running economy as a determinant of long-distance race performance. The runner with poor economy (1) requires a higher $\dot{V}O_2$ (approximately 10 ml kg^{-1} min^{-1}) to maintain a given running speed than the runner with good economy (4). Such a realistic difference in running economy (refer to Figure 4.11)

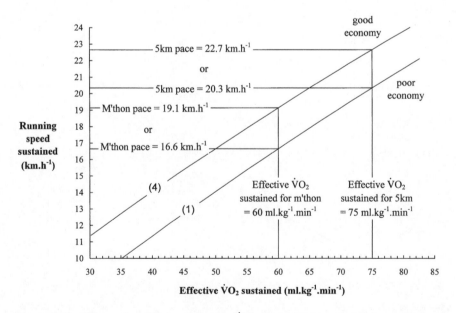

Figure 4.12. Effect of a difference in the $\dot{V}O_2$ demand for race pace running on performance in a 5 km and a marathon race

will have a dramatic effect on performance, translating into a 1.5 min advantage in a 5 km race (i.e. 13:13 vs 14:47) and a 20 min advantage in a marathon race (i.e. 2:13:00 vs 2:33:00). In contrast, Figure 4.13 emphasises how two runners who may be evenly matched at one distance can perform very differently at another distance if their running speed–$\dot{V}O_2$ relationships have different slopes. In Figure 4.11, the running speed– $\dot{V}O_2$ relationship for runner (2) has a *steeper* slope than that for runner (3). In presenting the same runners in Figure 4.13, a shallow slope on a line relating running speed to $\dot{V}O_2$ (Figure 4.11) is equivalent to a steep slope on a line relating the effective $\dot{V}O_2$ sustained to the running speed sustained. Thus, it is possible for two runners who have similar marathon race times (i.e. 2:21:30) to have 5 km race times which differ by 40 s (i.e. 13:42 vs 14:21) purely as a consequence of the different slopes of their respective running speed–$\dot{V}O_2$ relationship (Figure 4.13). For the same reason two runners may have the same 5 km race times but substantially different marathon race times.

The important point to note from the above discussion is that it is the running economy at race pace that will determine performance in a given event. That is, specialist 5 km runners need to have good running

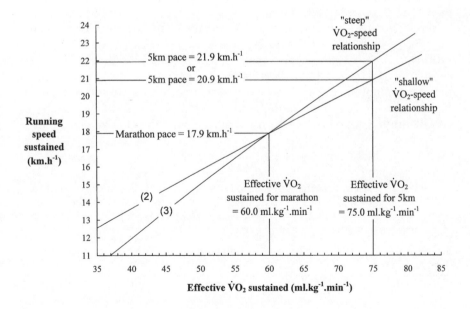

Figure 4.13. Effect of a difference in the slope of the $\dot{V}O_2$–running speed relationship on performance in a 5 km and a marathon race

economy at 5 km race pace, whilst specialist marathon runners need to have good running economy at marathon race pace. A runner who has a *steep* running speed–$\dot{V}O_2$ relationship (Figure 4.11) will have relatively good running economy at slow speeds but relatively poor running economy at fast speeds. Conversely, a runner with a *shallow* running speed–$\dot{V}O_2$ relationship will have relatively poor running economy at slow speeds but relatively good running economy at fast speeds. It is unlikely, therefore, that it will be possible for a runner who has a very steep running speed–$\dot{V}O_2$ relationship to have good economy at 5 km race pace. If such a runner was unable to reduce the slope of this relationship with training, there would be a strong argument to suggest that they should consider moving up to a longer distance event.

PHYSIOLOGICAL DETERMINANTS OF LONG-DISTANCE RUNNING PERFORMANCE

As was the case in Chapter 3 for middle-distance running performance, a model describing the inter-play between the physiological determinants of long-distance running performance, as well as the potential environmental and tactical determinants, can be developed (Figure 4.14).

Similar to the situation for middle-distance running performance, the influence of any one of the determinants detailed in Figure 4.14 on the estimated long-distance race time may also be calculated. Table 4.3 presents data from which the relative importance of each determinant may be evaluated. The influence on performance of a 10% improvement in each factor has been independently estimated. It is important in completing these analyses that the magnitude of the change is evaluated

Table 4.3. Percentage effect on estimated race time of a 10% improvement in $\dot{V}O_{2max}$, $\dot{V}O_2$ kinetics, sustainable %$\dot{V}O_{2max}$, anaerobic capacity and running economy in 5, 10, 21.1 and 42.2 km events

Race distance (km)	$\dot{V}O_{2max}$	$\dot{V}O_2$ kinetics	% $\dot{V}O_{2max}$ sustained	Anaerobic capacity	Running economy
5	7.3	0.4	2.3	0.5	7.5
10	7.5	negligible	6.7	negligible	7.5
21.1	7.8	negligible	7.8	negligible	7.5
42.2	8.0	negligible	8.0	negligible	7.5

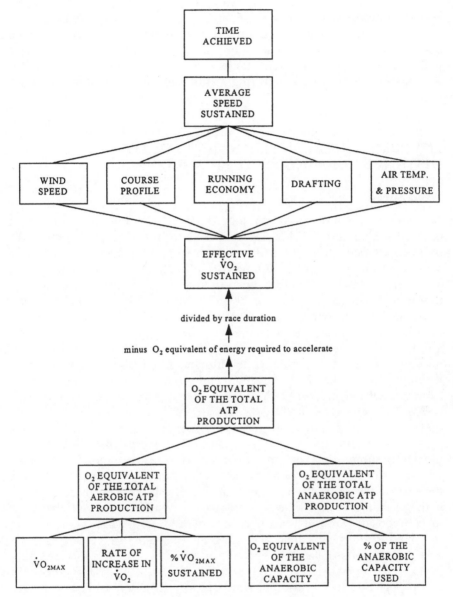

Figure 4.14. A model of long-distance running performance

against the maximum that could occur within physiological trainable limits (refer to Chapter 5).

Thus, a 10% increase in $\dot{V}O_{2max}$ and running economy would have a significant effect on race performance for all long-distance running events. Whereas a 10% improvement in the $\%\dot{V}O_{2max}$ sustained during an event will have an increasing influence on performance as race distance increases. Improvements in $\dot{V}O_2$ kinetics and anaerobic capacity will result in small improvements in race time during 5 km events, but will have a negligible effect during 10 km, half-marathon and marathon events.

ENVIRONMENTAL DETERMINANTS OF LONG-DISTANCE RUNNING PERFORMANCE

Wind Speed

The effect of wind speed on long-distance running performance is difficult to quantify. This issue was addressed with reference to middle-distance running performance in Chapter 3, in which comparisons were made between running into a head wind and running with a tail wind. The increase in oxygen uptake of running into a wind was found to be twice as large as the decrease in oxygen uptake when running with the wind (Davies 1980). This might be explained by the fact that athletes running with the wind will require energy to provide a braking force at the end of each flight phase, whilst athletes running into the wind will be braked by the increased air resistance. Thus, running into a head wind might be seen as more efficient than running with a tail wind. Moreover, the difference between the increase in $\dot{V}O_2$ associated with running into a head wind and the decrease in $\dot{V}O_2$ associated with running with a tail wind becomes greater as the wind speed increases. This seems reasonable, as a greater braking force would be provided by a stronger head wind, whilst a runner would need to provide a greater braking force when they had a strong tail wind. The practical implication of these findings is that a runner will not be able to accelerate sufficiently *with* the wind to compensate for the time that they would lose when running *into* the wind. This means that, assuming all else remains equal, performance in any long-distance event will always be worse on a windy day in comparison with a calm day and this decrease in performance will be proportional to the average wind speed encountered by the runner.

Course Profile

The effect of a 'hilly' course on long-distance running performance is analogous to the effect of relative wind speed and direction. The increase in $\dot{V}O_2$ observed when an athlete runs uphill is greater than the decrease in $\dot{V}O_2$ observed when they run downhill at the same combination of speed and gradient (Davies 1980). Similar to running with the wind, the athlete running downhill has to supply energy to provide a braking force at the end of each flight phase, but uphill running is like running against the wind, the athlete being braked by the resistive force of gravity. Thus, running uphill was seen as a more efficient activity than running downhill.

The implication of these findings is that a runner will not be able to accelerate sufficiently on downhill sections of a hilly course in order to compensate for the time they will lose on uphill sections. Once again assuming that if all else remains equal, long-distance running performance will always be worse on a hilly course in comparison with running on a flat course. This conclusion is supported by the work of Staab, Agnew and Siconolfi (1992), who compared running performance during two simulated 'races' staged on a treadmill. In one of the races the treadmill gradient was maintained at a zero gradient throughout the race. Whilst the other race incorporated both an uphill section (5 min at +5% grade) and a downhill section (5 min at −5% grade). The addition of a 'hill' was associated with a 2.6% decrease in performance, which would be equivalent to a 46 s increase for the 10 km race time of a typical long-distance runner. Thus, long-distance running performance will decrease when competing over a 'hilly' course in comparison with a flat course and it would be reasonable to suggest that the increase in race time would be proportional to the gradient of the hills a runner encounters.

Air Temperature

Chapter 3 described the interrelationship between air density, temperature and the air resistance encountered by a runner. You will recall that air density decreases as temperature increases, so air resistance will also decrease. From this discussion it was concluded that middle-distance race performance would be better on a warm day in comparison with a cold day. However, the situation is more complicated for a long-distance runner, where heat storage by the runner will become a major problem. This issue will be discussed in greater detail in Chapters 7 and 9. In brief, the human body is relatively inefficient; indeed the transfer of energy from metabolism into mechanical work is at best only about 25% efficient. The remaining 75% of energy is degraded in the form of heat, which must be removed from the body to allow normal physiological functioning to be maintained. The processes involved in this heat removal become less effective as the air temperature increases. It is likely that the potential gains associated with a relatively high air temperature (i.e. decreased air resistance) outweigh the potential losses (i.e. excessive heat storage) in middle-distance events. However, for long-distance races the potential losses would outweigh the potential gains, where excessive heat storage would be associated with impaired performance (Craig and Cummings 1966). This is particularly likely as long-distance races will be completed at slower speeds in comparison with middle-distance events, so that the influence of air resistance on race performance will be proportionately less.

Air Pressure

The impact of air (barometric) pressure on long-distance running performance is similar to the previously described effect on middle-distance running performance; the lower the air pressure, the less the air resistance and the better the potential race performance. However, there is an inverse relationship between the air resistance encountered by a runner and their average running speed. Therefore as the average race pace decreases with increasing race distance, the influence of air resistance on long-distance race performance becomes relatively unimportant.

TACTICAL DETERMINANTS OF LONG-DISTANCE RUNNING PERFORMANCE

Drafting

Drafting was discussed in Chapter 3, in which it was suggested that the benefit gained by a following runner was inversely proportional to their distance behind the lead runner. The minimum attainable distance between two runners decreases with decreasing running speed, so a long-distance runner would be able to run very close behind a lead runner in comparison with a middle-distance runner. Therefore a long-distance runner might reduce the air resistance they encounter by 50% (cf. 40% reduction in air resistance by a middle-distance runner; Kyle 1979).

If a runner was able to draft behind a competitor for the entire race, 5 km race performance would be improved by as much as 34 sec, or 4%. Adopting similar race tactics for the other long-distance events would result in a 3.7% (1.07 min) improvement in 10 km race time; a 3.3% (2.17 min) improvement in half-marathon race time and a 2.9% (4.10 min) improvement in marathon race time. Clearly drafting can have a significant effect on race performance in any long-distance event, but the relative influence of drafting decreases as race distance increases because the average running speed is slower.

Pacing Strategy

Pacing has not been included in Figure 4.14 as the tactical awareness of a runner is very hard to quantify. It is important to note that the best long-distance running performances are usually achieved when the time taken to complete the first half of the race is either equal to, or slightly greater than, the time taken to complete the second half. This pacing strategy appears to be optimal for all long-distance race events. For example, when Haile Gebrselassie ran 12:39.36 to set a new world record for the 5 km event in June 1998, the first half of the race was completed in 6:22.78 (i.e. 50.4% of the total time) and the second half was completed in 6:16.58. Similarly, in lowering the 10 km world record to 26:22.75 also in June 1998, Gebrselassie completed the first 5 km in 13:11.53 and the second 5 km in 13:11.22.

Tracking a long-distance runner's pacing strategy during the marathon becomes more complicated, as such events are often 'place to place' races. This means that runners may spend longer running into the wind or up a hill in one half of the race in comparison with the other half of the race. Nevertheless, when Renaldo Da Costa ran 2:06:05 in the 1998 Berlin Marathon to set the present world record, the first half of the race was completed in 64.42 min (i.e. 51.3% of the total time) and the second half a staggering 3.3 minutes quicker. Similarly, when Tegla Loroupe ran 2:20:47 to set a new women's world record in the 1998 Rotterdam Marathon, she covered the first half of the race in 70.2 min (i.e. 49.9% of the total time) and the second half in 70.6 min.

From the above discussion of pacing during long-distance events from 5 km through to the marathon, it is evident that the best runners achieve their best performances by maintaining a relatively constant race pace. In modern track and road competitions when an elite long-distance runner makes an attempt to establish a new world record, pacemakers are employed to control the pace during the first half of the race. Such a luxury is not normally available to the majority of runners and in the absence of this assistance a long-distance runner must be able to judge their own pace accurately. Furthermore, they must ensure that realistic targets are set and that they adhere to their predetermined race schedule. A mistake that is commonly made by runners, especially during the longer distance events such as the marathon, is to start too fast. Race performance will generally be less than optimal when a runner starts too fast and if a runner starts much too fast, the adverse effect on performance will be dramatic.

Overview: Maximising Long-Distance Running Performance

This chapter has considered data consistent with a typical long-distance runner to illustrate various aspects of the physiology of long-distance running performance. This approach is useful in linking physiological data with actual race performances, but it can also prove to be misleading. It should be emphasised that the model of a typical long-distance runner, similar to the typical middle-distance runner, is a theoretical construct. In reality, there is no such athlete as a typical runner.

For example, the differences between middle–long distance runners and specialist marathon runners have been discussed from both a physiological perspective and a performance perspective. However, both runners would be generally categorised as long-distance runners. Increasingly elite and club runners are specialising at one, or possibly two, distances with the 'all-round runner' becoming a less common athlete. The extent of this specialisation means that the feat of Emile Zatopek, winning gold medals for the 5 km, 10 km and marathon at the 1952 Helsinki Olympic Games, is unlikely to be repeated in the modern era. Moreover, it could be argued that there are now four distinct types of long-distance runner, each specialising in only one or two distances: the 3/5 km runner; the 5/10 km runner; the 10 km/half-marathon runner; and the marathon runner.

The 3/5 km Runner

This runner would compete often in 3 and 5 km track races, but would compete rarely, if at all, over 10 km. The Kenyan runner Daniel Komen would fall into this category. In the last few years, he has broken world records in both 3 and 5 km events.

The 5/10 km Runner

This runner would compete often in 5 or 10 km track events. They might occasionally compete over 3 km, but would rarely run on the road and are unlikely to race in events longer than 10 km. A runner of this type would be the Ethiopian Haile Gebrselassie, who has broken the 5 and 10 km world records several times each in recent years.

The 10 km/Half-Marathon Runner

This runner would compete often over 10 km on the track and on the road, as well as in half-marathon events on the road. They might also compete occasionally over 5 km on the track, usually at specific times or for specific reasons during their pre-season or season's training. Paul Tergat from Kenya would be an example of a 10 km/half-marathon runner. He has held the world record for the 10 km and the half-marathon events simultaneously in the last few years.

The Marathon Runner

At the extreme of long-distance running (as distinct from ultra-distance running) runners tend to specialise in one event. A marathon runner would compete fairly regularly in half-marathon and 10 km events, but the only distance at which they would expect to excel would be the marathon. The Spanish runners Martin Fiz, who was the 1996 European Champion and Abel Anton, the 1997 World Champion, are currently two of the best examples of specialist marathon runners.

Physiological Characteristics of the Different Types of Long-Distance Runner

A 3/5 km runner would be expected to have a substantial anaerobic capacity and a high $\dot{V}O_{2max}$. Consistent with any long-distance runner, a 3/5 km runner would be expected to show good race pace running economy (where race pace for these runners would be fast in relation to other long-distance runners), and they might also be expected to exhibit a relatively shallow running speed–$\dot{V}O_2$ relationship (Figure 4.11). A 3/5 km runner would be able to sustain a high relative exercise intensity for the duration of a 3 or 5 km race, but would not be able to maintain this race pace for events of a longer duration. This is because their high anaerobic capacity would maintain a high rate of anaerobic energy production during the shorter events. However, the %$\dot{V}O_{2max}$ that they would be able to sustain would be relatively low and therefore they would be unable to maintain a very high rate of aerobic energy production during the longer events. This low sustainable %$\dot{V}O_{2max}$ might be due to a lower ratio of type-I to type-II muscle fibres, a relatively low mitochondrial density within these fibres and a relatively low capillary density in their leg muscles. As a consequence, it is also likely that the lactate threshold of a 3/5 km runner would occur at a relatively low %$\dot{V}O_{2max}$.

In contrast, the marathon runner would be expected to have a relatively small anaerobic capacity and might also have a relatively low $\dot{V}O_{2max}$. This low $\dot{V}O_{2max}$ would be compensated for by sustaining a high %$\dot{V}O_{2max}$ (and therefore a high relative exercise intensity) for the duration of the marathon. Their leg muscles would comprise mainly type-I fibres with a high mitochondrial content, which would receive a good oxygen supply via a dense network of blood capillaries. These characteristics would allow marathon runners to sustain a high relative exercise intensity for the duration of a race without accumulating blood lactate (i.e. the lactate threshold would occur at a high $\%\dot{V}O_{2max}$). Finally, a marathon runner would show good running economy at marathon race pace and as this would be a relatively slow pace in comparison with a 3/5 km runner, they might be expected to have a steep running speed–$\dot{V}O_2$ relationship (Figure 4.11).

The 3/5 km runner and the marathon runner are at opposite ends of the long-distance running continuum and their physiological characteristics therefore represent the extremes of a continuum of such characteristics. For example, anaerobic capacity and $\dot{V}O_{2max}$ would be higher in a 3/5 km runner than in a 5/10 km runner, who in turn would have a higher anaerobic capacity and $\dot{V}O_{2max}$ than a 10 km/half-marathon runner, who in turn would have a higher anaerobic capacity and $\dot{V}O_{2max}$ than a marathon runner. Similarly the slope of the running speed–$\dot{V}O_2$ relationship would be steeper in a 5/10 km runner than in a 3/5 km runner, but this slope would be steeper in a 10 km/half-marathon runner than in a 5/10 km runner and steeper still in a marathon runner. Finally, the $\%\dot{V}O_{2max}$ at which the lactate threshold occurs would be higher in a 5/10 km runner than in a 3/5 km runner, but this percentage would be higher in a 10 km/half-marathon runner than in a 5/10 km runner and, once again, higher still in a marathon runner.

Can a Good Middle–Long Distance Runner Become a Good Marathon Runner?

Presently, there is much speculation over the potential success of Haile Gebrselassie when he eventually decides to move up to the marathon distance. His record of achievement pays testament to his pre-eminence as a long-distance runner. No successful marathon runner, past or present, has run below 27 min for a 10 km event, yet Gebrselassie has run 26:22.75! This has fuelled predictions that he will run 2:05.00, or even 2:04.00, on his marathon debut. Similar predictions have been made for Paul Tergat, whose best time for the 10 km event is 26:27.85.

This chapter has provided evidence to suggest that the best 5/10 km runner will not necessarily become the best marathon runner. For example, if Gebrselassie has a shallow running speed–$\dot{V}O_2$ relationship, his running economy at marathon race pace might not be good enough for him to dominate at this longer distance. Similarly, it may be that one of the reasons behind his success in 5 and 10 km events is that he is able to sustain a high relative exercise intensity for these events by virtue of a large anaerobic capacity. However, this would not allow him to sustain a high relative exercise intensity for the duration of a marathon. It is not known to what extent the ability of a marathon runner to sustain a high relative exercise intensity reflects their genetic endowment on the one hand and adaptation to long-distance training on the other. One possible determinant of the relative exercise intensity sustained would be the proportion of slow twitch fibres in a runner's leg muscles, which is generally considered to be a genetically defined trait. Thus, it is possible that even if Gebrselassie trains specifically for the marathon, he will not be able to sustain a high enough relative exercise intensity for the duration of a marathon race to allow him to be as successful at this longer distance as he has been at 5 and 10 km.

If the relevant physiological data (i.e. anaerobic capacity, running speed–$\dot{V}O_2$ relationship and $\%\dot{V}O_{2max}$ at which the lactate threshold occurs) were available for Gebrselassie, it would be possible to make an informed estimate of the time he would be able to achieve for a marathon. Without access to such data, it would be very difficult to endorse the predictions that have appeared in the popular running press with respect to his future running potential. The above discussion would suggest that not even the 'greats', such as Gebrselassie, can readily excel across the distance divide.

KEY POINTS

- The anaerobic energy contribution to long-distance running performance is small in the 5 and 10 km events and negligible in the half-marathon and marathon events.
- As the rate of oxygen uptake is relatively constant for the majority of long-distance events, $\dot{V}O_2$ kinetics is unimportant as a determinant of performance.
- Although the anaerobic capacity is not generally an important determinant of long-distance performance, it can play an important role in the 5 km event for which it can make a significant contribution to the relative exercise intensity sustained.
- The actual $\%\dot{V}O_{2max}$ sustained is an important determinant of long-distance race performance and tends to be highest in specialist marathon runners.
- Running economy is also important, and must be evaluated at race pace. Runners who are economical at marathon race pace may be uneconomical at 5 km race pace.
- $\dot{V}O_{2max}$ is an important determinant of long-distance running performance, but marathon runners may compensate for a lower $\dot{V}O_{2max}$ than

5–10 km runners by sustaining a higher %$\dot{V}O_{2max}$.

- Improving $\dot{V}O_{2max}$ and running economy will have a significant effect across all long-distance events, whereas improving the %$\dot{V}O_{2max}$ sustained will have a greater effect as race distance increases.
- Long-distance performance will always be worse on a windy day and/ or on a hilly course compared with a calm day and/or on a flat course.
- Drafting can significantly reduce the $\dot{V}O_2$ demand to run at race pace and could improve long-distance performance by 3–4%.
- Pacing strategy is important across all long-distance races. These are usually run at a relatively constant pace with the second half normally being slightly quicker than the first.

Chapter 5

Training for Middle and Long-Distance Running

David M. Wilkinson

INTRODUCTION

The foundations to world record breaking performances are rooted in the attributes we inherit from our parents and to be successful at the international level, runners need the necessary physiological qualities and the ability to develop these qualities through appropriate physical training. Unfortunately, not everyone has the genetic potential to be an elite middle or long-distance runner but all healthy athletes possess the ability to improve their performance through an effective training programme. This Chapter discusses training strategies, which focus upon the key physiological determinants identified in Figures 3.14 and 4.14, to improve middle and long-distance running performance.

PRINCIPLES OF TRAINING: PRESCRIBING THE TRAINING OVERLOAD

Training adaptations are achieved through systematically *overloading* the physiological systems which determine (or limit) performance. The training overload can be defined in terms of duration, frequency and intensity. *Training duration* defines the length of each training session and can be easily prescribed and monitored with a stopwatch. *Training frequency* refers to the number of sessions completed within a particular time period and again can easily be prescribed and monitored by counting the number of sessions performed. *Training intensity* defines the quality of the training effort, which presents more of a problem for the runner to define. The obvious answer in prescribing training intensity would be to monitor running speed during a session, but changes in terrain and environmental conditions make the link between running speed and relative exercise intensity highly variable. These, coupled with the practical problems of measuring the distance means that except for track sessions, speed *per se* may not be the best method of setting and monitoring training intensity.

There are a number of comparable approaches to expressing relative exercise intensity and these are presented in Table 5.1. Technical Box 5.1 describes a common approach, based upon a runner's individual heart rate response, that is increasingly used to prescribe and monitor training intensity.

TECHNICAL BOX 5.1

Monitoring Training Intensity by Heart Rate

One approach to prescribing training intensity that has gained widespread appeal is based on a runner's heart rate response to increasing running speeds. The training intensity continuum can be divided into discrete zones, where each zone is linked to a particular level or intensity of training. Each training level is defined in terms of a corresponding heart rate range, the specific range for each runner being based on their individual blood lactate response to incremental exercise. Figure 5.1 illustrates a typical heart rate and blood lactate response to increasing exercise intensity (running speed), where heart rate increases linearly and blood lactate concentration increases curvilinearly.

Blood lactate provides a measure of a runner's relative exercise intensity, where the increase in blood lactate concentration indicates greater physical stress on the muscles. At *easy* to *moderate* relative exercise intensities, the blood lactate concentration remains relatively low. This indicates a relatively low stress on the muscles and therefore this intensity might be maintained for several hours. This is *level-1* and, and on the example given in Figure 5.1, would correspond with a heart rate range of less than approximately $150\,\text{b}\,\text{min}^{-1}$. Level-1 sessions should be used for low-intensity recovery training, where the running pace is relaxed and comfortable. The majority of prolonged, steady state, *moderate* intensity endurance training would be performed at *level-2* (or low-intensity endurance training). Level-2 training would equate to a heart rate range of 150–165 b min^{-1} in the example, where the blood lactate concentration is just starting to increase indicating a moderate level of stress on the muscles. A runner would have to concentrate to maintain the required relative exercise intensity during level-2 training, but would be able to hold a conversation with a training partner. *Level-3* training is at a *hard* relative exercise intensity, performed within the heart rate range of 165–185 b min^{-1}, and represents the upper limit of endurance training (or high-intensity endurance training). This type of training is relatively stressful on the muscle; it is therefore best performed as tempo runs of 20–40 min of hard effort or long intervals of 5–15 min with variable recovery, where the emphasis is on maintaining *form* and running smoothly. *Level-4* training corresponds to the rapidly increasing section of the blood lactate–running speed relationship and a heart rate range greater than 185 b min^{-1}. Training at this relative exercise intensity is associated with a rapid accumulation of blood lactate and high levels of fatigue in the runner; therefore these relatively stressful sessions can only be performed as short intervals (less than 3 min). At these high exercise intensities, heart rate will only give an indication that the runner is in the level-4 zone, but heart rate can be usefully used to monitor recovery. The emphasis of level-4 training is quality; it differs from level-3 training in that the intervals are shorter and the intensity is higher, and the rest periods are longer to allow more complete recovery and good running form to be maintained. Table 5.1 provides a general guide for equating the various forms of expressing exercise intensity used throughout this book.

This approach to prescribing training intensity generally allows the training stress to be carefully monitored, but it is not without its limitations. Excessive fatigue, illness, anxiety and environmental conditions will all affect the heart rate training response. Therefore a runner should familiarise themselves with the 'feel' of a session when in a healthy, rested state and use heart rate monitoring more as an indicator of their state of fatigue. Heart rates that are more than 5–10 b min^{-1} higher or lower than what would normally be expected for a standard training session may indicate inadequate recovery and/or illness, and appropriate action should be taken immediately.

MAXIMUM OXYGEN UPTAKE

The $\dot{V}O_{2max}$ of most elite male distance runners is greater than 70 ml kg^{-1} min^{-1} (Noakes 1991) and elite female distance runners is greater than

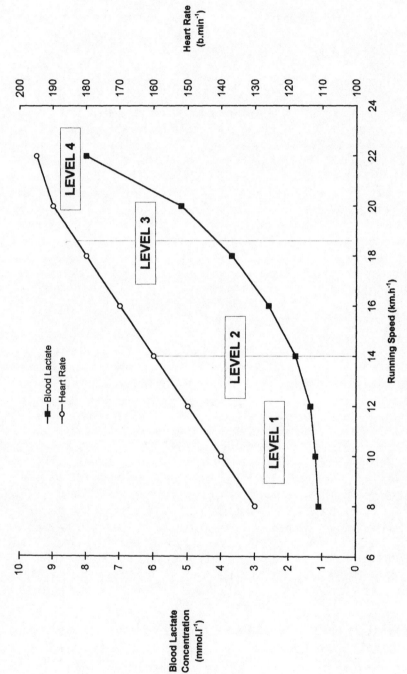

Figure 5.1. The heart rate and blood lactate response to progressive exercise

Table 5.1. A guide to equating the expression of exercise intensity

Type	Level	%$\dot{V}O_{2max}$	%heart rate$_{max}$	Race pace
Easy	1	< 65	< 75	Ultra-marathon
Moderate	2	70–85	75–85	< Marathon–1/2 marathon
Hard	3	90–100	85–95	10–5 km
Intervals	4	> 100	> 95	3000–100 m

65 ml kg^{-1} min^{-1} (Costill 1986). The importance of a high $\dot{V}O_{2max}$ is high-lighted in Figure 5.2, which illustrates the now familiar running speed–$\dot{V}O_2$ relationship. Clearly, the higher a runner's $\dot{V}O_{2max}$, the higher their peak running speed, and the better their endurance performance poten-tial. From Figure 5.2 it is evident that a runner with a $\dot{V}O_{2max}$ of 50 ml kg^{-1} min^{-1} would not be able to complete a marathon in 2:30:00 (required average speed 16.88 km h^{-1}) as this would demand a rate of oxygen uptake of 55 ml kg^{-1} min^{-1}. If it is assumed that a typical long-distance runner would sustain 80% $\dot{V}O_{2max}$ for the duration of this race (Maughan and Leiper 1983), a $\dot{V}O_{2max}$ of 69 ml kg^{-1} min^{-1} would be required by a runner to complete the marathon in the target time.

It is tempting to speculate that the best middle and long-distance runners would have the highest $\dot{V}O_{2max}$. However, $\dot{V}O_{2max}$ is only one of the key physiological factors determining the average speed sustained during a race (Figures 3.14 and 4.14). A high $\dot{V}O_{2max}$ gives a runner the

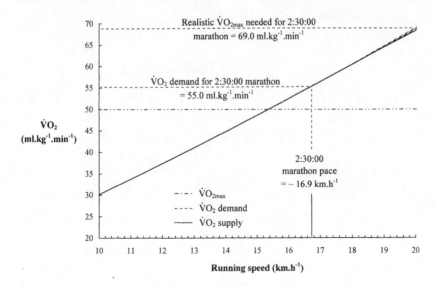

Figure 5.2. Schematic representation of the $\dot{V}O_2$ demand for a 2:30.00 marathon

potential to be an elite middle and long-distance runner, but actual performance will reflect their sustainable $\%\dot{V}O_{2max}$, running economy and, where appropriate, anaerobic capacity. Nevertheless, the trainability of $\dot{V}O_{2max}$ is an important consideration, where a 10% improvement was shown in Chapters 3 and 4 to improve significantly middle and long-distance race performance. It is therefore not surprising that increasing $\dot{V}O_{2max}$ is frequently a principal target of many endurance training programmes.

TECHNICAL BOX 5.2

Transfer of Oxygen from the Atmosphere to Muscle

The limitations to $\dot{V}O_{2max}$ were briefly discussed in Chapter 4. The journey of oxygen from the atmosphere to the mitochondria in cells involves a complex series of linked events. The first event in this oxygen chain involves ventilation, the movement of atmospheric air in and out of the lungs. Oxygen is transferred from the lungs into blood by the process of diffusion, the net movement from a high concentration to a low concentration. Oxygen is then carried in blood, mainly bound to haemoglobin, where the heart is responsible for pumping the blood around the body. On arrival at the capillary bed in tissue, oxygen diffuses from its relatively high concentration in blood, through the capillary walls and into the muscle fibres. This process is facilitated by the presence of myoglobin, an iron-containing pigment present in muscle that acts as a transient oxygen store, which has a stronger affinity for oxygen in comparison to haemoglobin. The final destination is the mitochondria, where oxygen is used in the aerobic production of energy.

LIMITATIONS TO MAXIMUM OXYGEN UPTAKE

The general consensus of the scientific community is that the major limitation to $\dot{V}O_{2max}$ is the pumping capacity of the heart (Poole and Richardson 1997). A number of studies have demonstrated that $\dot{V}O_{2max}$ can be increased if the supply of oxygen to the tissue is artificially increased through blood doping (Spreit *et al.* 1986, Robertson *et al.* 1982) or by increasing the percentage of oxygen in inspired air (Knight *et al.* 1993). This suggests that *peripheral* muscle would be able to use more oxygen if the heart was able to increase *central* supply. Thus, training to improve $\dot{V}O_{2max}$ should target the pumping ability of the heart or maximum cardiac output. Cardiac output is determined by both the stroke volume of the heart (i.e. volume of blood ejected from the heart per beat) and the heart rate (i.e. number of times the heart beats per minute). A normal value for resting cardiac output would be $5.0 \, l \, min^{-1}$, increasing to $25–35 \, l \, min^{-1}$ during high-intensity exercise. However, values in excess of $40 \, l \, min^{-1}$ have been reported in elite distance runners. The maximum heart rate of a typical distance runner normally falls between approximately $175–190 \, b \, min^{-1}$ and is not significantly changed by training. Therefore, improvements in cardiac output and hence $\dot{V}O_{2max}$, must come from an increase in heart size which in turn would increase stroke volume.

TRAINING TO INCREASE HEART SIZE

High-volume training consisting of prolonged, moderate to hard intensity sessions appears to be the best stimulus for promoting an increase in heart volume (George, Wolfe and Burggraf 1991). The size of this stimulus, and therefore the resulting degree of adaptation, is related to the intensity and duration of the training overload. As exercise intensity increases, stroke volume increases (Gledhill, Cox and Jamnik 1994) and this will increase the tension and stretch on the walls of the heart during filling. The result over the long term will be enlargement of the heart and improved contractility of heart muscle. However, Wagner (1996) highlighted the importance of muscle capillarisation as an often ignored limitation in the chain of oxygen delivery to the muscle. It appears that the interaction between cardiac output and muscle capillary density dictate the amount of oxygen that can be delivered to muscle (i.e. central limitation).

OTHER LIMITATIONS TO MAXIMUM OXYGEN UPTAKE

At sea-level, $\dot{V}O_{2max}$ is thought to be limited by central oxygen delivery to the muscle. However, Chapter 9 illustrates how the reduced partial pressure of atmospheric oxygen at altitude and hence the reduced pressure of oxygen in a runner's lungs, blood and muscle, can also limit $\dot{V}O_{2max}$. There have been a number of reports recently which suggest that nearly 50% of healthy, well-trained male endurance athletes ($\dot{V}O_{2max}$ greater than $70 \, ml \, kg^{-1} \, min^{-1}$) may show a fall in the oxygen concentration of blood leaving the lungs at sea level when exercising at relative intensities above 80% $\dot{V}O_{2max}$ (Powers, Martin and Dodd 1993).

This is called exercise-induced hypoxaemia and suggests that the lungs in these highly trained athletes may not function optimally in loading the blood with oxygen. As the presence of exercise-induced hypoxaemia has important implications for runners training and competing at both altitude and at sea level, its identification should be an important part of any physiological assessment procedure. Identification can be achieved non-invasively using exercise-validated pulse oximeters, which simply clip to the runner's finger or ear lobe and estimate the saturation of haemoglobin in blood with oxygen[1] (Powers *et al.* 1988, Powers *et al.* 1989).

Runners who experience exercise-induced hypoxaemia need to focus their training on improving the transfer of oxygen from the lung into blood (i.e. their lung diffusion capacity), rather than maximal cardiac output. Indeed, high cardiac outputs in these runners may well be partly responsible for the lower than normal oxygen levels in blood leaving the lung. A high cardiac output will be associated with a high rate of blood flow around the capillaries of the lungs, which will therefore reduce the time that red blood cells have to pick up oxygen (Dempsey 1987, Powers *et al.* 1989). It is possible that lung diffusion capacity is not very trainable and may therefore set the upper limit for $\dot{V}O_{2max}$ in some elite runners. This might explain why some elite endurance athletes possess a relatively low $\dot{V}O_{2max}$, despite their high volume training, and compensate by sustaining a high %$\dot{V}O_{2max}$ with good running economy (e.g. Derek Clayton, the former world record holder for the marathon who was discussed in Chapter 4).

GUIDELINES FOR TRAINING TO IMPROVE MAXIMUM OXYGEN UPTAKE

The intensity, frequency and duration of training interact to influence $\dot{V}O_{2max}$ (Wenger and Bell 1986). In relatively untrained individuals, improvements in $\dot{V}O_{2max}$ are associated with all training intensities above 50% $\dot{V}O_{2max}$, but the greatest gains are made in untrained and trained individuals at exercise intensities of 90–100% $\dot{V}O_{2max}$. This is consistent with the argument presented above, where high-intensity (level-3/4) training maximally taxes heart stroke volume and provides the optimal stimulus for cardiac enlargement. These types of training sessions could be 35–40 min in duration, comprising 3–6 min intervals at speeds equivalent to 3–5 km race pace. Alternatively, Wenger and Bell (1986)

---

[1]Oxygen is essentially carried in the blood bound to haemoglobin (97%) and dissolved in plasma (3%). Under normal circumstances the blood will almost be fully oxygenated, with all the binding sites of haemoglobin being full and plasma being completely saturated.

found that longer duration runs ($>$ 45 min) at lower intensities (level-2) may elicit similar effects, possibly by targeting muscle capillarisation to increase oxygen delivery. The interaction between intensity and duration of endurance training in already well-trained runners is not clear and scientific studies examining long-term training in elite runners are scarce.

TECHNICAL BOX 5.3

Case Study of Steve Scott

The American 1500 m (3:31.96) and mile (3:49.68) record holder in 1981, Steve Scott, was followed over the nine month competitive season during which he broke these records (Conley *et al.* 1984). After a break following the end of the previous season during which he had only performed 'light distance workouts', his $\dot{V}O_{2max}$ in September 1980 was 74.4 ml kg^{-1} min^{-1}. In December he included one long (1000–5000 m) interval session per week on top of the distance workouts he had been performing. This was supplemented by shorter (200–600 m) intervals in January. February was devoted to regular indoor racing with longer distance sessions interspersed. By March 1981, his $\dot{V}O_{2max}$ had increased to 77.2 ml kg^{-1} min^{-1}. For the next three months he returned to running 100 miles week^{-1}, incorporating some short intervals and weight training. His $\dot{V}O_{2max}$ by the end of the season was reported as 80.1 ml kg^{-1} min^{-1}, a 7.3% increase from an already impressive initial value. Thus, both interval training and a large volume of long slow distance training may be associated with increases in $\dot{V}O_{2max}$ in previously well-trained runners.

Not all well-trained runners will show a significant change in $\dot{V}O_{2max}$ during a season. Svedenhag and Sjödin (1985) observed that $\dot{V}O_{2max}$ was relatively stable over a season in Swedish endurance athletes, improving only when these athletes performed high-intensity interval (level 3/4) training. Further evidence to support high-intensity interval training for improving $\dot{V}O_{2max}$ comes from the fact that middle-distance runners, who perform a much higher percentage of their total training volume as high-intensity intervals tend to have a higher $\dot{V}O_{2max}$ than marathon runners. Daniels and Daniels (1992) reported that elite middle–long distance (M–LD) (5/10 km) runners had a higher $\dot{V}O_{2max}$ (77 ml kg^{-1} min^{-1}) than elite marathon runners (74 ml kg^{-1} min^{-1}). Pollock (1977a) and Svedenhag and Sjödin (1984) also reported higher $\dot{V}O_{2max}$ values in elite M–LD runners (78 ml kg^{-1} min^{-1}) in comparison with marathon runners (74 ml kg^{-1} min^{-1}). It is possible that this is simply a result of natural selection, where runners with a higher $\dot{V}O_{2max}$ are naturally successful and therefore self-select the shorter events, rather than a difference in the respective training strategies *per se*.

With respect to recommendations for training volume to increase $\dot{V}O_{2max}$, four sessions per week of high-intensity (level 3/4) training appears to be optimal in runners with a $\dot{V}O_{2max}$ in the region of 50 ml kg^{-1} min^{-1} (Wenger and Bell 1986). Costill (1986) monitored two marathon runners returning to fitness after a six-month lay-off. Gains in $\dot{V}O_{2max}$ plateaued with a weekly running mileage of 60–90 miles. This is not to suggest that every runner should immediately start to train 60–90 miles each week! Most runners spend a number of years gradually increasing their mileage, allowing their bodies time to adapt and cope with the stresses imposed by high-volume training. Indeed, sudden increases in weekly mileage will inevitably result in excessive tissue damage (Chapter 7), injury or overtraining.

In summary, whilst a high training volume (up to 90 miles week^{-1}) is undoubtedly important for developing and maintaining a high $\dot{V}O_{2max}$, and is commonly undertaken by well-trained distance runners, the addition of short high-intensity interval sessions may maximise training gains. These sessions should be designed to stress stroke volume maximally, where this high level of stress should be maintained for the maximum possible time. Intervals should not be too short (i.e. less than 3 min), as time is required for cardiac output to reach maximal values. However, if the intervals become too long (i.e. greater than 6 min), runners may not be able to perform, both physically or mentally, enough intervals to achieve the required overload. The recovery between intervals should be relatively short (i.e. less than 1 min); oxygen uptake would drop if the permitted recovery was too long and a greater demand would be placed on anaerobic energy production at the start of each new interval. Table 5.2 summarises the general principles of training to improve $\dot{V}O_{2max}$.

Table 5.2. General training principles for improving $\dot{V}O_{2max}$

Mode	Intensity (%$\dot{V}O_{2max}$)	Duration (min)	Reps	Rest (min)	Frequency (sessions per week)
Continuous	60–80	30–120	–	3–6	
Intervals	90–100	3–6	5–10	0.5–1.5	1–4

POTENTIAL IMPROVEMENTS IN MAXIMUM OXYGEN UPTAKE

The potential for improving $\dot{V}O_{2max}$ is commonly reported as limited in trained athletes. Improvements of 15–40% have been reported in previously sedentary individuals, although increases as great as 93% have been observed (Pollock 1973). These values are consistent with those reported for Jim Ryun, a former American mile record holder (3:51.1). Ryun's trained $\dot{V}O_{2max}$ of 81.0 ml kg^{-1} min^{-1} fell to 65 0 ml kg^{-1} min^{-1} after a year's lay-off and rose again to 78.3 ml kg^{-1} min^{-1} with two years retraining, a change over the three years of around 20% (Daniels 1974). This example would support the fact that there is a finite level of improvement in $\dot{V}O_{2max}$ (Daniels 1974, Daniels *et al.* 1978b, Svedenhag and Sjödin 1985), which may be genetically limited, physiologically limited (i.e. lung diffusion capacity or maximal cardiac output) or simply reflect the type of training being performed. Evidence of a genetic component in determining $\dot{V}O_{2max}$ was presented by Bouchard (1990). Ten pairs of identical twins were monitored during a 20 week endurance training programme. Each twin in a pair similarly improved in $\dot{V}O_{2max}$ following the programme, though there was considerable variation in responses between sets of twins with increases in $\dot{V}O_{2max}$ ranging from 0–12%.

As well as training strategies, both gender and age influence $\dot{V}O_{2max}$. The values of $\dot{V}O_{2max}$ of female athletes are typically 8–12% lower than male athletes (Wilmore and Costill 1994). This is mainly due to a smaller heart size (and therefore smaller stroke volume), lower blood volume, lower blood haemoglobin concentrations and higher body fat percentage in comparison with male athletes. Independent of gender, ageing is associated with a reduction in $\dot{V}O_{2max}$ equivalent to 1% per year after the age of 30, though this trend can be minimised by continued training (Pollock *et al.* 1987).

RUNNING ECONOMY

Running economy is defined in Chapter 3 as the $\dot{V}O_2$ required to run at a given speed and is commonly expressed in units of millilitres of oxygen per kilogramme body weight per minute (ml kg^{-1} min^{-1}). The importance of running economy was highlighted by Conley and Krahenbuhl (1980), who reported that over 65% of the variability in race performance in trained runners of similar ability (average 10 km time of 32:06) and similar $\dot{V}O_{2max}$, was accounted for by differences in running economy. Thus, successful distance runners usually possess better running economies than less successful runners. This view would be supported by the data presented in Chapter 4 on the marathon world record holder Derek Clayton. Clayton (2:08:33 marathon) had a running economy of 45 ml kg^{-1} min^{-1} (Costill *et al.* 1971b) whilst treadmill running at 16 km h^{-1}.

However, examination of the limited information published on elite distance runners suggests that this is not always the case. The running economy of 53 ml kg^{-1} min^{-1} reported for Craig Virgin (2:10:26 marathon) and 50 ml kg^{-1} min^{-1} reported for Jim Ryun (mile 3:51.1)[2] at 16 km h^{-1} (Noakes 1991) are not very different from the running economy of 50–55 ml kg^{-1} min^{-1} reported in untrained individuals. This raises the possibility that, similar to $\dot{V}O_{2max}$, running economy may be largely genetically determined, with limited scope for improvement through training.

FACTORS INFLUENCING RUNNING ECONOMY

Training

When running economy was expressed in ml kg^{-1} km^{-1} (see Chapter 6), there were no differences between elite male and elite female distance runners at relative (% $\dot{V}O_{2max}$) exercise intensities typically sustained in races up to marathon distance (Daniels and Daniels 1992). These workers also reported that running economy (when expressed in ml kg^{-1} km^{-1}) increases as exercise intensity increases for most elite middle and long-distance runners. Nevertheless, 25% of runners showed no increase in economy and 9% actually showed a decrease, demonstrating that running economy is relative exercise intensity dependent. The majority of runners displaying these atypical responses were 800 and 1500 m specialists and may have demonstrated an adaptation in response to their higher average training pace. Although no differences were found in running economy between middle and long-distance runners at marathon race pace, the middle-distance runners were more economical at 800 and 1500 m race pace (Daniels and Daniels 1992). This may reflect that both groups will perform some of their training at marathon race pace (i.e. long slow distance running), but only the middle-distance runners will perform a significant part of their training at 800 and 1500 m race pace, suggesting the possibility that training adaptations to running economy are intensity specific.

---

[2]World mile record in 1967.

Short-term (i.e. less than 3 months) training programmes have usually failed to show improvements in running economy, which are evident following longer ones (i.e. 3 months to 5 years) for elite runners (Conley *et al.* 1984, Svedenhag and Sjödin 1985, Morgan and Craib 1992, Jones 1998). However the magnitude of these improvements are relatively small (i.e. 3 to 9%), considerably smaller than the 20–30% differences in running economy observed in trained runners of similar ability (Morgan and Daniels 1994). This would give further support to the view that training can have some impact on running economy, but a large component will reflect inherited physiological and/or biomechanical factors.

Age

The oxygen cost of running is reported to decrease by about 25% from seven years of age through to 18, even in the absence of any formal running training (Daniels *et al.* 1978a, MacDougall *et al.* 1983). Prolonged running training during these developing years appears to further enhance those improvements which naturally occur with ageing. Interestingly, those runners who have good running economy when young also have good running economy when older (Krahenbuhl, Morgan and Pangrazi 1989), further supporting a strong genetic influence. Improvements in running economy with age have been attributed to decreasing metabolic rate, increases in oxygen diffusion capacity in the lung evident from a decrease in ventilatory equivalent for oxygen, and more advantageous stride mechanics as limb lengths increase (Krahenbuhl and Williams 1992).

Stride Mechanics

The relationship between running mechanics and running economy has been extensively reviewed (Williams 1990, Anderson 1996) but with limited practical outcomes. There is a range of mechanical variables that show some relationship with running economy, though these relationships do not appear to be general for all groups of runners, or for all individuals within a defined population group. Most of the mechanical variables identified such as height, mass distribution around the lower leg and narrow pelvis cannot be modified by training. Furthermore, even if running mechanics are improved it does not necessarily follow that running economy will be improved (Messier and Cirillo 1989). Thus, at present there are no clear guidelines for modifying running mechanics in order to improve running economy (Williams 1990).

Muscle Fibre Recruitment

One of the more obvious differences between poor and elite runners is the apparent inherent ease of an elite runner's action. They seem to *flow* over the track or road with minimal effort, although there are exceptions to this rule who have gone on to achieve international success. It is possible that through years of endurance training, elite runners develop and refine their *skill of running*, so that only the essential running muscles are recruited. This would reduce the oxygen cost incurred due to the recruitment of antagonist and/or excessive recruitment of stabilising muscles, thus reducing the total oxygen cost of running and improving running economy.

This view is supported by the observation that runners completing a high training volume greater than approximately 75 miles week^{-1} show better running economy than lower volume runners (Svedenhag and Sjödin 1985, Scrimgeour *et al.* 1986). However it should be borne in mind that self-selecting groups rather than running economy might be the common factor in such a cross-sectional analysis. In other words those runners with good economy may be more successful at long-distance races than those with poor economy, and therefore participate for this reason. High training mileage will not be appropriate for all middle and long-distance runners. Indeed, for some runners, economy may be improved through performing high-intensity interval (level-3/4) training (Conley *et al.* 1981, Conley *et al.* 1984, Sjödin, Jacobs and Svedenhag 1982). The argument is made in Chapters 3 and 4 that it is running economy at race pace that is important in determining middle and long-distance running performance, not running economy *per se*. For example, Daniels and Daniels (1992) reported that specialist 800 and 1500 m runners tend to have relatively better economy at higher running speeds in comparison with specialist marathon runners, as evident in a lower slope in their running speed–$\dot{V}O_2$ relationship (refer to Chapter 4). Thus, middle-distance runners who race at higher speeds must focus upon improving their economy during race pace running. This would be supported by the need to improve the skill of *race pace* running with respect to a runner's specialist event and the requirement of a specific training overload in order to elicit the desired training adaptation.

Muscle Fibre Type

Type-I (slow twitch) muscle fibres may be more oxygen efficient in producing energy through aerobic metabolism in comparison with type-II (fast twitch) muscle fibres (Schantz and Henriksson 1987, Gaesser and Poole 1996). Therefore runners who possess a high percentage of type-I fibres may produce more energy for a fixed amount of oxygen, compared to runners with a higher percentage of type-II fibres, at running speeds where the majority of type-I fibres are recruited. In agreement, marathon runners, who possess a greater slow twitch muscle fibre type profile than middle-distance runners (Costill Fink and Pollock 1976, Howald 1982), tend to be more economical than middle-distance runners at marathon speeds (Svedenhag and Sjödin 1994, Daniels and Daniels 1992). The current scientific consensus suggests that training cannot bring about transformations between type-I and type-II fibres. However, you will recall from Chapter 4 that type-II fibres can be further differentiated into type-IIa and type-IIb fibres, where type-IIa fibres have a greater oxidative capacity or greater ability to use oxygen to produce energy than type-IIb fibres. Endurance training has been associated with sub-type fibre trans-formations (Andersen and Henriksson 1977, Howald 1982). Thus, a general fast twitch to slow twitch (i.e. type-IIb to type-IIa) transformation may account for the small changes in running economy reported follow-ing many years of endurance training (Williams and Cavanagh 1987).

Elastic Energy Storage

The ability of muscle and tendon to store elastic energy during the ground impact phase of the running cycle (i.e. elastic energy storage) and return this energy during the take-off phase, is an important determinant of the oxygen cost of running. Indeed, there would be an estimated 30–40% increase in this oxygen cost if elastic energy storage did not contribute to the running action (Cavagna, Komarek and Mazzoleni 1971), but there is considerable variation between individuals in their abilities to store and effectively utilise elastic energy (Williams and Cavanagh 1983). This may partly explain some of the variation in the running economy of middle and long-distance runners, especially at higher running speeds where the greater impact forces (and hence potentially greater elastic energy storage) might become more important. A link between the ability to store elastic energy in the muscle during jumping and running economy has been demonstrated by Bosco, Mon-tanari and Ribacchi (1987).

GUIDELINES FOR TRAINING TO IMPROVE RUNNING ECONOMY

Running economy can be improved through training (Bailey and Pate 1991), although the precise nature of the adaptations are not clear. As skill learning is usually specific to the training activity, run training at race pace to improve running economy seems a logical step. This strategy is supported by the observations that adaptations leading to improved running economy at long-distance race pace (e.g. fibre type transformations) may be different from those improving running economy at middle-distance race pace (e.g. elastic energy storage).

Middle-distance runners will have to perform this training as intervals to ensure that an appropriate volume of high-intensity training can be achieved. Rest periods should be long enough to ensure that good *form* is maintained during the interval repetitions. Saltin *et al.* (1995a) also speculated that running on rough and varied terrain might explain the excellent running economies usually found in young Kenyan athletes. As such, hill running (sprints) might be included as part of a training strategy for improving running economy in middle-distance runners.

The shorter event (i.e. 5/10 km) long-distance runners could use long intervals or continuous running to achieve an appropriate training overload, whilst specialist marathon runners are likely to perform this training as long slow-distance running (Table 5.3). The total volume of training performed at race pace seems to be an important factor for improving running economy, especially in the longer races. As a consequence, rapid short-term improvements are unlikely and this form of training to improve running economy should be viewed as part of a long-term training strategy.

ANAEROBIC ENERGY PRODUCTION

The importance of anaerobic energy production to optimising middle-distance running performance was highlighted in Chapter 3 (Table 3.1). The methods adopted to improve the runner's ability to produce energy anaerobically are specific to each event. Increasing the *rate* at which energy can be generated anaerobically (i.e. anaerobic power) will im-

Table 5.3. General training principles for improving running economy

Event	Intensity	Duration (min)	Reps	Rest	Frequency (sessions per week)
800/1500 m	Race pace	1–3	5–10	~ Full recovery	1–3
3/5/10 km	Race pace	5–30	1–5	~ Full recovery	1–3
21.1/42.2 km	Race pace	30–120	–	–	1–3

prove 400 m performance, but not distances of 800 m or longer. This is because the anaerobic capacity (i.e. the total amount of energy generated anaerobically) of a middle-distance runner is unlikely to be exhausted in events lasting less than one minute (Medbo *et al.* 1988). Consequently, specialist 400 m runners need to include training sessions designed to increase their rate of anaerobic energy production, whilst this type of training may not be necessary for runners who compete in the longer events. Similar to 400 m race performance, the rate of anaerobic energy production is also a very important determinant of 100 and 200 m sprint performance. This similarity would explain why the training of 400 m runners tends to bear more resemblance to the training of 200 m sprinters than that of 800 m middle-distance runners. It may also explain why the 400 m is often considered more as an extended sprint rather than a middle-distance event, and why athletes such as Michael Johnson can compete successfully at international level in both the 200 and 400 m.

In contrast, as anaerobic capacity may be exhausted in middle-distance events of 800 m and longer, runners in these events should focus on training to improve the total amount of energy they are able to produce anaerobically (i.e. anaerobic capacity).

GUIDELINES FOR TRAINING TO IMPROVE ANAEROBIC ENERGY PRODUCTION

Training to Improve Anaerobic Power

The rate of anaerobic energy production during middle-distance running is dependent upon the rate of energy production from glycolysis (refer to Technical Box 5.4). This, in turn, is highly dependent upon the concentration of enzymes that catalyse glycolysis within the muscle fibre. Maximal sprinting is likely to produce maximal activation of these enzymes and therefore provide an appropriate stimulus for adaptations to increase the enzymes' activity and hence the rate of glycolysis. Peak activation of the glycolytic enzymes may not be attained until after 5 s of sprinting. Therefore, very short sprints (i.e. less than 5 s) may rely too heavily on high-energy phosphates (ATP and phosphocreatine) stored in the muscle for anaerobic energy production and have limited effect on maximising the rate of glycolysis.

The optimal duration of maximal sprints for improving the rate of anaerobic energy production is somewhere between 5–30 s. As maximal speed is required to maximally activate glycolysis, rest periods between sprint repetitions should be long enough to allow full recovery. Rest periods of 3–5 min would allow most of the high-energy phosphates stores to be replenished (Harris *et al.* 1976, Casey *et al.* 1996). Shorter rest periods may achieve full recovery from 5–10 s sprints, but would not be long enough to ensure full recovery from longer sprints. Recovery will be improved by active recovery such as walking or light jogging between sprints. The number of repetitions is determined by the number of sprints that a runner is able to perform before sprinting form is lost, but would usually be between 3–10 repetitions. A summary of the guidelines for improving anaerobic power are given in Table 5.4.

TECHNICAL BOX 5.4

Anaerobic and Aerobic Glycolysis

Fuels for anaerobic energy production include adenosine triphosphate (ATP), phosphocreatine (PCr) and carbohydrates (glucose and glycogen) stored in the muscle fibre. Glycolysis is a sequence of reactions converting glucose to pyruvate: anaerobic glycolysis may occur when there is inadequate oxygen present and pyruvate is converted to lactate; aerobic glycolysis refers to the process whereby carbohydrates are completely metabolised to carbon dioxide and water when there is adequate oxygen available in the muscle.

Training to Improve Anaerobic Capacity

The factors influencing the total amount of energy produced anaerobically in a sedentary (untrained) individual and an elite 800 m runner are given in Table 5.5. There are limited data on the anaerobic capacities of elite middle-distance runners, however a value of over $100 \, \mathrm{ml \, kg^{-1}}$ has been reported for the Kenyan 800 m runner Benson Koech who ran 1:43 in 1994, which may partly explain his exceptional time despite a modest $\dot{V}O_{2max}$ of $72 \, \mathrm{ml \, kg^{-1} \, min^{-1}}$ (Saltin *et al.* 1995a).

The oxygen stored, by combining with haemoglobin in blood and

Table 5.4. General training principles for improving anaerobic power

Event	Intensity	Duration (s)	Reps	Rest (min)	Frequency (sessions per week)
Middle distance	Maximal	5–30	3–10	> 2–5 (full recovery)	2–4

Table 5.5. Estimated relative contribution of the components of anaerobic capacity for a sedentary individual and an elite 800 m runner (Adapted from Saltin 1990 and Medbo *et al.* 1988)

Component of anaerobic capacity	Contribution to anaerobic capacity			
	Sedentary	Elite	Sedentary	Elite
	($ml\,kg^{-1}$)		(% of total)	
O_2 bound to haemoglobin and myoglobin	5	6	11	6
High-energy phosphates (ATP and phosphocreatine)	14	19	31	19
Glycolysis (carbohydrate to lactate)	26	75	58	75
Total	45	100	100	100

myoglobin in muscle, and the high-energy phosphate pool of ATP and phosphocreatine, are relatively unaffected by training, and would therefore only have a small influence on increasing anaerobic capacity (Table 5.5). The greatest potential for improving a runner's anaerobic capacity lies in enhancing energy production from glycolysis. The muscle's stores of carbohydrate in the form of glycogen, which provides the fuel for glycolysis during intensive exercise, are not depleted during a single bout of exercise at a running speed equivalent to middle-distance race pace. However, the processes by which energy is generated anaerobically from carbohydrates during intensive exercise result in the production of lactate and associated hydrogen ions. It is the hydrogen ions which, in turn, are thought to both inhibit energy metabolism and disrupt further muscle contraction. Hence, the limitation to anaerobic energy production appears to be the muscle's ability to neutralise (buffer) the hydrogen ions associated with lactate formation.

Thus, training to improve anaerobic capacity should be maximal or near maximal to overload the processes involved in glycolysis and the subsequent management of lactate and hydrogen ions. Maximal intensity interval runs should be between 20–45 s in duration; near maximal runs will allow a longer period of exercise of 45–120 s before fatigue, although more moderate intensity intervals are also effective (Weston *et al.* 1997). The rest periods between intervals should allow some running form to be maintained, but should not be long enough to allow full recovery and therefore the training stimulus on muscle buffering capacity will be maintained. Walking or light jogging can be performed during the rest periods, but should be kept to a minimum to limit lactate clearance from the muscles and therefore again maintain the training stimulus. A summary of the guidelines for improving anaerobic capacity are given in Table 5.6.

Not all the hydrogen ions associated with lactate production are buffered within the muscle fibre. One approach that the muscle adopts in managing hydrogen ions, so muscle contraction is maintained, is by rapidly transporting lactate and hydrogen ions out of the muscle. The blood capillary network surrounding type-II (fast twitch) muscle fibres, which have a high glycolytic capacity, facilitates the removal of lactate and hydrogen ions to other organs such as the heart and type-I muscle fibres that are suited to lactate metabolism. Therefore, prolonged endurance training which results in some type-II muscle fibres taking on more slow twitch fibre characteristics, including an increase in capillary density, may be an alternative strategy to increasing muscle buffering capacity for improving anaerobic capacity.

General Considerations for Improving Anaerobic Energy Production

The training adaptations contributing to improved anaerobic energy production (i.e. improved glycolytic enzyme levels and buffering capacity) occur within the muscle fibre. Consequently, any training benefits will only be realised if the muscle fibres recruited during training are the same as those recruited during race performance. This reinforces the concept of *training specificity* and highlights the importance of running training to improve anaerobic energy production in middle-distance runners.

POTENTIAL IMPROVEMENTS IN ANAEROBIC ENERGY PRODUCTION

Adaptation in glycolytic enzyme levels and muscle buffering capacity appear to occur fairly rapidly, taking between a few days to a few weeks

Table 5.6. General training principles for improving anaerobic capacity

Event	Intensity	Duration (s)	Reps	Rest (min)
Middle distance	Maximal	20–45	3–10	1–2 (limited)
	Near-maximal	45–120	2–8	3–8 (limited)
	High ($\geq$ 10 km race pace)	300	6–8	1 (limited)

of training (Weston *et al.* 1997). Tabata *et al.* (1996) reported that six weeks of sprint training (i.e. 7–8 repetitions at 170% $\dot{V}O_{2max}$ for 20 s with 10 s rest) improved anaerobic capacity by 28% (i.e. 60 to 77 ml kg^{-1}). Maximum oxygen uptake was also increased by 15% (i.e. 48 to 55 ml kg^{-1} min^{-1}), confirming that high-intensity interval training can be useful in terms of both aerobic and anaerobic training adaptations.

Medbo and Burgers (1990) compared two different six week training programmes (three days per week) designed to improve anaerobic energy production during running. The first was designed to improve anaerobic power, where 8×20 s efforts with approximately 5 min walk/jog recovery were performed. The intensity was prescribed to exhaust volunteers in 35–40 s if the speed had been maintained for this duration (i.e. 165% $\dot{V}O_{2max}$ or 200 m race pace). The runs used approximately 43% of pre-training anaerobic capacity during each 20 s repetition. The second training programme was designed to improve anaerobic capacity, where 3×120 s efforts with approximately 8 min walk/jog recovery were performed. The intensity was prescribed to exhaust volunteers in 3.0–3.5 min if the speed had been maintained (i.e. 116% $\dot{V}O_{2max}$ or 1500 m race pace). The runs used approximately 74% of pre-training anaerobic capacity during each 120 s repetition. Both training programmes increased anaerobic capacity by 10%, but notably there were no differences in anaerobic power despite the different relative training intensities.

Interestingly, altitude exposure has been shown to improve both muscle buffering capacity (Saltin *et al.* 1995b) and anaerobic capacity in middle-distance runners (Chapter 9). This was despite the fact that the training performed at altitude was relatively low intensity, aerobic training. This observation would therefore support the inclusion of altitude training in the preparation of both sprint/power and endurance athletes.

The degree of anaerobic training adaptation with long-term (years) specific training is presently not known. However, as sprint-trained athletes typically report maximal accumulated oxygen deficit (MAOD)[3] values that are approximately 30–50% higher than sedentary (untrained) or endurance-trained athletes (Medbo and Burgers 1990). This would support either a genetic limitation (natural selection) or that long-term training may have an influence.

The interaction between anaerobic capacity and both attainable %$\dot{V}O_{2max}$ and $\dot{V}O_2$ kinetics was discussed in Chapters 3 and 4. Increasing the anaerobic capacity allows the middle-distance runner to sustain a higher relative exercise intensity during a race, speeding $\dot{V}O_2$ kinetics and increasing the final %$\dot{V}O_{2max}$ attained. Improvements in middle-

---

[3]Refer to Chapter 6 for a description of MAOD as a measure of anaerobic capacity.

distance performance would be greater than predicted from the increases in anaerobic capacity alone, although this effect would be small for race distances over 5 km (Table 4.3).

THE RATE OF INCREASE IN OXYGEN UPTAKE ($\dot{V}O_2$ KINETICS)

Chapter 4 highlighted the minimal effect of improving $\dot{V}O_2$ kinetics on long-distance race performance. Although its impact on middle-distance race performance is also relatively small, training to increase $\dot{V}O_2$ kinetics is a sound strategy for specialist 800 m runners as improvements in race performance will be greater than those calculated for increases in $\dot{V}O_2$ kinetics alone. Faster $\dot{V}O_2$ kinetics would result in a high %$\dot{V}O_{2max}$ being attained by the end of the event. There seems little purpose in training to increase $\dot{V}O_2$ kinetics in the longer middle-distance events as the 1500 and 3000 m events are already run at approximately 100% $\dot{V}O_{2max}$ (Table 3.2; Chapter 3).

GUIDELINES FOR TRAINING TO IMPROVE $\dot{V}O_2$ KINETICS AT RACE PACE

The most suitable training for improving $\dot{V}O_2$ kinetics at race pace is likely to be high-intensity interval running (level-4). This form of training will increase anaerobic capacity (Table 5.6), allowing a higher relative exercise intensity to be sustained during a race, which will increase $\dot{V}O_2$ kinetics and the %$\dot{V}O_{2max}$ attained during an 800 m event. It is also the ideal form of training for increasing $\dot{V}O_{2max}$ (Table 5.2), and the more rapid increase in cardiac output at the onset of exercise due to an increased stroke volume may be a factor responsible for the improvement in $\dot{V}O_2$ kinetics with this form of training.

TRAINING TO IMPROVE %$\dot{V}O_{2max}$ SUSTAINED IN LONG-DISTANCE RUNNING (5/10 km)

The majority of trained long-distance runners can sustain a rate of oxygen uptake that is very close to $\dot{V}O_{2max}$ for the duration of a 5 km (98% $\dot{V}O_{2max}$) and a 10 km (92.4% $\dot{V}O_{2max}$) race. Therefore the potential for the %$\dot{V}O_{2max}$ sustained to increase during these events is relatively small. The theoretical maximum increase possible for the typical long-distance runner given in Chapter 4 is 7.6% in a 10 km race, which resulted in a

6.7% improvement in race performance. However, as a 7.6% increase in the %$\dot{V}O_{2max}$ attained in a 10 km race is unrealistic, most runners can only maintain a running speed at $\dot{V}O_{2max}$ for approximately 5–10 min and to focus training on improving this component of 5 and 10 km performance is probably unwise. Nevertheless, training to increase the relative exercise intensity sustained for the duration of these events could be achieved by improving anaerobic capacity (Table 5.6).

TRAINING TO IMPROVE %$\dot{V}O_{2max}$ SUSTAINED IN LONG-DISTANCE RUNNING (HALF-MARATHON AND MARATHON)

In contrast to the 5 and 10 km events, the %$\dot{V}O_{2max}$ sustained during a half-marathon and marathon are typically below 100% $\dot{V}O_{2max}$, so a significant increase in the total amount of energy produced aerobically over the duration of the race should be associated with an increase in race performance. The main fuels for aerobic energy production are carbohydrates (stored as muscle glycogen, liver glycogen and blood glucose) and fats (both intramuscular and blood borne fat stores). The maximum rate at which fats can supply energy can only sustain running speeds equivalent to 50–60% $\dot{V}O_{2max}$; therefore faster race pace runs require an increasing contribution from carbohydrates. Although this contribution from carbohydrates is provided aerobically in the first instance[4], there is an increasing contribution from anaerobic (glycolysis) carbohydrate metabolism as running speed exceeds approximately 85% $\dot{V}O_{2max}$.

Relying upon anaerobic energy sources to meet the total energy demand in longer distance running is counterproductive. The energy yield from the anaerobic breakdown of carbohydrate is only 9% of that derived from aerobic carbohydrate breakdown. Thus anaerobic carbohydrate metabolism is associated with a rapid depletion of the muscle's finite carbohydrate stores, which will become an issue of greater concern as race distance increases. Hence the %$\dot{V}O_{2max}$ sustained in long-distance races is dependent upon the capacity of the muscle to use oxygen and its capacity to produce energy aerobically at a high rate. This is referred to in Chapter 4 as the oxidative capacity of muscle, and is influenced by the proportional distribution of type-I fibres in the muscle (Ivy *et al.* 1980),

---

[4]The fate of pyruvate as the end-point of glycolysis in part depends on the availability of oxygen in the muscle, which in turn is dependent upon the exercise intensity of a runner relative to their $\dot{V}O_{2max}$.

the number of mitochondria in each fibre, the activity of aerobic enzymes and the muscle capillary density (Coyle *et al.* 1991).

Training to increase the $\%\dot{V}O_{2max}$ that a runner can sustain for the duration of a long-distance race should therefore be geared towards improving the oxidative capacity of muscle (Coyle *et al.* 1988). Large training volume seems important for the initial adaptation to the $\%\dot{V}O_{2max}$ sustained during long-distance races, but after a few years of extensive endurance training (i.e. greater than 57 km week^{-1}) performance improvements may reflect improvements in running economy rather than improvements in $\%\dot{V}O_{2max}$ sustained (Scrimgeour *et al.* 1986). However, the larger the training volume, the lower the average training speed is likely to be. It is important that the weekly volume does not become so high that the average training speed is well below race pace, for as discussed previously, changes in running economy require speed-specific training. This might also explain the steeper slope on the running speed–$\dot{V}O_2$ relationship for marathon runners, who tend to be more economical than middle-distance runners at slow speeds but less economical at fast speeds (Daniels and Daniels 1992). Training strategies to increase the $\%\dot{V}O_{2max}$ sustained for long-distance running would be similar to those outlined in Table 5.3 for increasing running economy in marathon runners, although the intensity may be less important than the duration of the training.

VARIABILITY IN $\%\dot{V}O_{2max}$ SUSTAINED DURING LONG-DISTANCE RACING

It is impractical to measure routinely the amount of oxygen consumed over a marathon in order to determine the actual $\%\dot{V}O_{2max}$ sustained for the duration of the race. Therefore the majority of scientific studies that have examined the $\%\dot{V}O_{2max}$ sustained during long-distance races have had to estimate this value. This is usually achieved by estimating the average $\dot{V}O_2$ supply from a runner's individually determined running speed–$\dot{V}O_2$ relationship (e.g. Figure 4.2) and expressing this estimated $\dot{V}O_2$ supply as a percentage of a treadmill-determined $\dot{V}O_{2max}$. However, Figure 4.2 also highlights the fact that this treadmill-determined $\dot{V}O_2$ supply does not equal the $\dot{V}O_2$ demand to run at race pace as it does not take into consideration the additional oxygen cost of overcoming air resistance in track/road running. The $\%\dot{V}O_{2max}$ determined from a treadmill running speed–$\dot{V}O_2$ relationship will progressively underestimate the actual $\%\dot{V}O_{2max}$ sustained as race speed increases above approximately 13 km h^{-1}, the speed where air resistance starts to make a significant impact on the total oxygen cost of running. It is therefore important to take into consideration this additional oxygen cost when comparing the $\%\dot{V}O_{2max}$ sustained by runners of differing ability.

An additional problem arises from the fact that $\%\dot{V}O_{2max}$ sustained decreases as race duration increases (Maughan and Leiper 1983). So as well as correcting for air resistance when comparing the $\%\dot{V}O_{2max}$ sustained in runners of different abilities, a correction should also be made for differing race durations. These two points are seldom acknowledged in the scientific literature.

The $\%\dot{V}O_{2max}$ sustained during a marathon varies between 60% $\dot{V}O_{2max}$ for 5:00:00 runners to approximately 80% $\dot{V}O_{2max}$ for 2:20:00 runners (Maughan and Leiper 1983, Sjödin and Svedenhag 1985). This value of 80% $\dot{V}O_{2max}$ for the faster runners is considerably lower than the 91% reported for Derek Clayton, the former marathon world record holder, who was able to sustain an exceptionally high $\%\dot{V}O_{2max}$. However, if the figure quoted for the 2:20:00 marathon runners is corrected for air resistance and for the difference in race times of 9%, their calculated value approaches 89% $\dot{V}O_{2max}$. Similarly, if the data reported by Sjödin and Svedenhag (1985) are corrected for air resistance and differences in race times, it becomes evident that elite, good and slow marathon runners who have undertaken some prolonged endurance training can sustain approximately the same $\%\dot{V}O_{2max}$ for the same duration of event.

The slow runners in the Sjödin and Svedenhag study had trained for 2.4 years and averaged 57 km week^{-1} compared to the elite runners who had be training for over 7 years and averaged 145 km week^{-1}. Untrained runners certainly sustain a lower $\%\dot{V}O_{2max}$ than trained runners if the differences in race time are taken into account, and so the change in $\%\dot{V}O_{2max}$ sustained may be a relatively early adaptation (i.e. less than 2 years) to prolonged endurance training. The ability to improve this $\%\dot{V}O_{2max}$ further with continued prolonged endurance training is not known. Stable values have been reported for elite middle and long-distance runners over the course of a season (Svedenhag and Sjödin 1985), and Daniels and Daniels (1992) reported that six out of eight elite female marathon runners sustained between 84.0 and 84.9% $\dot{V}O_{2max}$, the remaining two runners sustaining 82.8 and 88.2% $\dot{V}O_{2max}$. However, it should be noted that although the average values for different groups of runners is similar when corrected for air resistance and race duration, there is still considerable variation between runners of a similar ability. Once again it is not clear whether this variability is genetic or a result of the training performed. The former seems likely as the change in $\%\dot{V}O_{2max}$ sustained after extensive endurance training appears relatively stable, but the volume of training performed is important.

As a postscript to the above discussion, the $\%\dot{V}O_{2max}$ estimates reported in the scientific literature are generally average values sustained during the race. It is important to remember that there may be substantial fluctuations around this average value in road races due to changes in terrain. Maron *et al.* (1976) directly measured oxygen uptake in two runners completing a marathon (2:38:00) and reported that 77% $\dot{V}O_{2max}$ was utilised during level running, compared with 68% $\dot{V}O_{2max}$ during downhill running and nearly 100% $\dot{V}O_{2max}$ during uphill running.

OVERTRAINING

Overtraining has be defined as an imbalance between training and the recovery process (Lehmann *et al.* 1997), and its prevalence is high in middle and long-distance runners. Morgan *et al.* (1987) reported that 65% of elite runners experienced staleness at some time during their competitive careers. It is usually caused by an increase in training volume and/or intensity, resulting in long-term (weeks to months) performance decrements in the absence of any medical condition (Budgett 1990). The ensuing collection of symptoms associated with overtraining are collectively referred to as overtraining syndrome (Lehmann, Foster and Keul 1993, Lehmann *et al.* 1997). Despite the growth in overtraining research over the last decade, there are currently no valid and reliable physiological or biochemical markers of impending overtraining. This is probably not surprising since prospective research studies designed to induce overtraining syndrome are difficult to perform and counterproductive for most athletes aiming to optimise performance. Difficulties also arise in defining the boundary between over-reaching and overtraining. Over-reaching is a short-term condition characterised by sub-optimal performance that is reversible with several days of rest or recovery training (Fry, Morton and Keast 1991). Over-reaching is frequently encountered by athletes who use a 'crash microcycle' as part of their training strategy (Fry, Morton and Keast 1992). This involves performing several days of hard training, with limited recovery time, to induce a high degree of stress on the body. The resulting adaptations are thought to be superior to those gained when more extensive recovery time is taken between training sessions. It has been suggested that over-reaching is an early stage of overtraining and long term performance decrements may result if adequate rest is not taken (Fry *et al.* 1991, Fry and Kraemer 1997). Therefore the key to preventing overtraining may lie in the identification of over-reaching. Table 5.7 identifies some of the practical symptoms that may accompany the onset of over-reaching and overtraining, although it is important to note that some runners may not show all of the symptoms listed and others may not show any, except impaired performance.

It is also important to reinforce that the only definitive symptom that

Table 5.7. General symptoms associated with over-reaching and overtraining in runners

Over-reaching	Overtraining
Impaired performance	Impaired performance
General state of excitation	General state of depression
Poor recovery after training	Poor recovery after training
Restlessness	Lethargy, apathy
Disturbed sleep (sweating)	Deep, undisturbed sleep
Weight loss	Stable weight
Increased resting heart rate	Decreased resting heart rate
Increased exercising heart rate	Decreased exercising heart rate
Slowed heart rate recovery	Rapid heart rate recovery
Increased illness rate	Increased illness rate
	Early onset of hypoglycaemia

has been reported in all over-reaching/overtraining studies is continued under-performance after an 'adequate' period of rest. Therefore training should be phased or periodised by combining periods of high and low training volume on a day by day, weekly, monthly and yearly cycle. Training progress should be closely monitored via performance during 'easy' phases within the training calendar. Any unexplained stagnation or deterioration in performance in the absence of a medical condition should always be carefully evaluated by the runner and coach. Over-reaching or overtraining should always be considered as **one** possible explanation for the loss of form. Recovery from over-reaching is usually achieved by extended rest (1–4 weeks), with or without light training. The recovery process from overtraining is less certain, with a very gradual return to training over a period of months being performed by the very few athletes who have documented their experiences.

TAPER TRAINING

In an effort to maximise the benefits from weeks of hard training, many endurance athletes reduce their training volume for a period of 5–21 days prior to important competitions. This process is often called tapering as the training volume progressively decreases or 'tapers' as the competition approaches. The effects of taper training on performance are well documented in swimming (Costill *et al.* 1985) and cycling (Martin *et al.* 1994) but the effects on middle and long-distance running performance are less clear.

Houmard *et al.* (1990) reported that reducing training distance by 70%

(from 81 km week^{-1}) for 21 days had no effect on 5 km time trial performance (16:30). Furthermore, McConell *et al.* (1993) found that if a similar reduction in training volume was accompanied by a reduction in training intensity to include only long slow distance running, 5 km time fell by 1.2% (from 16:36). The importance of training intensity was reinforced by Shepley *et al.* (1992) who found that time to exhaustion at 1500 m race pace was only improved (22%) when training intensity remained high, despite a large reduction in training distance from 80 km week^{-1} to 7.5 km week^{-1} in a 7 day taper. Houmard *et al.* (1994) confirmed that a similar 7 day taper involving an 85% reduction in training volume, all performed as 400 m intervals at 5 km race pace, improved 5 km performance by 3%. This improvement was not just a function of a decreased total training volume, as runners following the same taper regimen on bicycles failed to modify 5 km running performance. Most of the improvement in the 5 km performance in the running taper group appeared to be a result of an improved running economy, reinforcing the specificity of training argument for both the mode of training performed and the intensity-specific adaptations required for improving running economy. One interesting finding from this last taper study was that many of the runners reported sore muscles as a result of the unaccustomed volume of high-intensity interval training (Chapter 7), despite improving performance. This could be avoided by gradually introducing some high-intensity interval work into the training programme in the weeks preceding the taper period.

A similar low-volume high-intensity taper regimen for longer distance runners may not have the same performance benefits. Wilkinson *et al.* (1997) reported that a 7 day taper had no effect on improving simulated half-marathon performance (1:24:29) or running economy. As most longer distance runners will perform a much greater volume of training near to race pace, high-intensity taper training may have its greatest effect on those athletes who spend the least amount of training volume at race pace. In addition, as many of the training adaptations that contribute to maintaining a high sustainable % $\dot{V}O_{2max}$ are training volume dependent, they may rapidly decrease with low-volume training or detraining (Klausen, Andersen and Pelle 1981). Although this may not be a major problem for the middle-distance runner, it will have an increasing effect as race duration increases in long-distance events as the capacity to sustain a high % $\dot{V}O_{2max}$ increases (Chapter 4). For the long-distance runner, a gradual reduction in training mileage would certainly reduce the training-induced muscle damage (Chapter 7) associated with prolonged endurance training and maximise the glycogen stores (Chapter 8) prior to competition. However the use of high-intensity intervals which may add to the degree of muscle damage appear unnecessary.

SUMMARY

It is important to remember that the methods of training presented in this chapter are only guidelines. Every runner has a different genetic potential for improvement and runners will adapt in different ways to identical training sessions. Unfortunately for the runner and coach, sports science is never going to be able to identify the *ultimate* training programme for a middle and long-distance runner. Clear guidelines have been given as to the type of training likely to produce the specific adaptations required to improve $\dot{V}O_{2max}$, $\%\dot{V}O_{2max}$, running economy, $\dot{V}O_2$ kinetics, anaerobic power and anaerobic capacity. However, sports science can measure each of these specific physiological components, enabling the runner and coach to identify appropriate training targets. Regular physiological monitoring throughout the season can assess the efficacy of a current training programme and provide guidance for setting future training targets (Chapter 6).

KEY POINTS

- Training adaptations are achieved through systematically overloading the body, with this overload being defined in terms of the intensity, duration and frequency of training.
- A high maximum $\dot{V}O_{2max}$ appears to be a pre-requisite for successful middle and long-distance running performance, and seems to respond to both high-intensity interval training and long slow distance training in different runners.
- The $\dot{V}O_{2max}$ of some elite runners may not be limited by central delivery of oxygen to the muscle, but by diffusion of oxygen across the lung (exercise-induced hypoxaemia). These runners may respond better to long slow distance training to further increase $\dot{V}O_{2max}$, as increasing cardiac output may only add to the problem of hypoxaemia.
- The determinants of a good running economy are not currently known. Increasing elastic energy storage in the muscles may be more important for improving economy in middle-distance runners, whilst changing muscle fibre type may be more important in long-distance runners.
- Improvements in running economy seem fairly small in comparison to the differences between good runners, suggesting a strong genetic influence. Changes that do occur appear to take a number of years and training to improve running economy should be viewed as a long-term strategy.
- Anaerobic capacity can be improved by performing short, high intensity intervals or a relatively brief spell (i.e. approximately two weeks)

at altitude.
- The %$\dot{V}O_{2max}$ sustained in the longer distance races is dependent upon the oxidative capacity of the muscle and responds to increasing training volume, although differences between already well-trained runners are small.
- Overtraining is of increasing concern amongst runners and care should be taken to include adequate rest on a regular basis as part of a sound training regimen.
- A low-volume interval taper programme prior to competition may improve performance in events of 5 km and less, but a more gentle reduction in training volume with little change in intensity may be a more appropriate strategy for long-distance runners.
- The most effective way to monitor the success of a training programme is by careful physiological monitoring, as the individual responses to any training programme are highly variable.

Chapter 6

Physiological Assessment of the Middle and Long-Distance Runner

David M. Wilkinson

INTRODUCTION

This chapter examines the issues involved in assessing the physiological determinants of middle and long-distance running performance with respect to optimising training. Notwithstanding that the ultimate test of a runner's fitness is competition itself, the benefits of physiological monitoring are two-fold. First, a race time will represent the collective product of all determinants underpinning performance, therefore making it impossible to identify the individual contributions of each determinant. This information is vital if training is to be tailored to address the specific weaknesses of a runner. Second, it is rarely practical to rely exclusively on scheduled race events to monitor training progression. It is doubtful that marathon runners would relish racing 42.2 km every time they wished to check that every- thing was progressing well!

Assessment of middle and long-distance runners can be undertaken using specialist equipment to measure the key physiological determinants of performance. This is frequently carried out by running on a motorised treadmill in a laboratory whilst expired air is collected and analysed to calculate the amount of oxygen being used. Simple performance-based tests that are dependent upon one or more of the key physiological determinants of middle and long-distance performance are also widely used, usually being performed in a gymnasium, on the track/road, or on a playing field.

PREPARATION BEFORE ASSESSMENT

Regardless of the venue for assessment there must be careful preparation by the runner and assessor to ensure that, as far as possible, the data obtained are influenced only by the physiological status of the runner and not any other potentially confounding variables. Issues that require attention include the following

- Environmental conditions (i.e. temperature, humidity and wind speed). These tend to be much less of a problem in a laboratory setting, especially in air-conditioned facilities. Ideal environmental conditions would include a stable environment at 16–18 °C, relative humidity between 40 and 60% and cooling fans to provide a controlled air flow for the runner.
- The running surfaces such as polished gym floor, tarmac or tartan track should be the same for repeated measurements, especially for shuttle-running tests where turning becomes more difficult if the surface is slippery.
- Footwear such as training shoes, racing flats, running spikes or even bare feet should be the same for repeated assessments.
- The nutritional, psychological and fatigue status of the runner is an important consideration. Have they just eaten their lunch? Do they need to get away early? Or, have they performed 10 × 800 m intervals at race pace the night before attending? The runner should only perform light training or rest in the preceding 48 hours before assessment and refrain from training during the day preceding assessment. A light, high carbohydrate meal should be consumed 2–4 hours before arriving at the assessment venue, during which consumption of alcohol and caffeine-containing beverages and food (e.g. Coca-Cola, chocolate, coffee, tea) should be minimised.

The purpose of any good assessment is to determine whether a runner has changed their physiological status, not whether the assessment process is different.

This chapter highlights some important issues to consider when performing a physiological test, so that the data is meaningful and can be used with confidence to design the optimal training programme. In addition, results reported in the scientific literature from a range of middle and long-distance runners will be summarised to allow comparison and identification of individual strengths and weaknesses within a physiological profile.

THE NATURE OF PHYSIOLOGICAL ASSESSMENT: WHAT TO ASSESS

As sports science has matured as a discipline, there is a considerable range of assessment procedures now available for monitoring trained athletes. However, a runner is only really interested in those factors that determine performance. The tests undertaken should assess $\dot{V}O_{2max}$, %$\dot{V}O_{2max}$ sustained, race pace running economy in both middle and long distance runners, $\dot{V}O_2$ kinetics, and anaerobic capacity in middle-distance runners.

ACCREDITATION OF PROFESSIONAL COMPETENCY

A physiological assessment can be both a stressful and an expensive experience. It is therefore essential that those performing the assessment are accredited to do so. This will ensure they adhere to a professional 'Code of Conduct'. Such a code will be concerned with the professional competence of a sports scientist as well as ethical issues and client confidentiality. In the United Kingdom, the process of laboratory and sports scientist accreditation is overseen by the British Association of Sport and Exercise Sciences (BASES).

Prior to any form of exercise test it is important that a runner completes some form of health appraisal. This is usually in the form of a check-list questionnaire, though it may be accompanied by a resting medical examination including body weight, height, blood pressure, electrocardiogram, lung function and blood screening. These procedures help to verify that the runner is *safe to exercise*.

LABORATORY-BASED PHYSIOLOGICAL ASSESSMENT

The following section presents general descriptions of the assessment procedures that might be adopted in monitoring middle and long-distance runners. Some of the tests must be completed in a prescribed order as information is required from a previous test to complete calculations in a subsequent test. Thus, test order for the physiological assessment of our typical middle or long-distance runner is: determination of capillary blood haemoglobin concentration (optional) and haematocrit (optional), lung function (optional), running economy, $\dot{V}O_{2max}$ (%$\dot{V}O_{2max}$ sustained could then be calculated using a recent race time) and for the middle-distance runner, anaerobic capacity. These tests may be performed on separate days.

Determination of Blood Haemoglobin Concentration

Haemoglobin (Hb) is the oxygen transporting component of red blood cells, so the concentration of haemoglobin in blood is an important determinant of oxygen transport to active tissues and an important determinant of middle and long-distance running performance. It is made up of four protein chains attached to a haem molecule containing ferrous iron. Low blood concentrations of haemoglobin may be indicative of an iron deficient diet, impaired dietary iron absorption from the gut or abnormal iron metabolism within the body.

The determination of haemoglobin concentration in capillary blood drawn from a prewarmed finger or ear, may result in a value that is slightly lower than the actual concentration in whole blood. The normal ranges for blood haemoglobin concentrations are: male runners 14–18 $g\,dl^{-1}$; female runners 12–15.5 $g\,dl^{-1}$.

If low haemoglobin concentrations are reported, the best course of action would be to consult a general practitioner to rule out any clinical cause before a nutritional solution is sought. A qualified sports dietician or sports nutritionist should be consulted if a dietary cause is suspected.

Middle and long-distance runners undergoing high-volume training tend to fall at the lower end of the normal range due to increases in plasma volume in response to training. Alternatively, low concentrations in trained runners (aside from a nutritional or absorption problem) might reflect red blood cell damage which is discussed in greater detail in Chapter 7. This has resulted in some controversy regarding the lowest values that should be tolerated before seeking medical advice. Many elite endurance athletes report concentrations well within this normal range. Martin and Coe (1997) reported that 15 elite male marathon runners (2:16:00) were well within the normal range with a mean value of 15.7 g dl^{-1}. Saltin *et al.* (1995a) similarly reported concentrations for a group of elite Kenyan (14.9 $g\,dl^{-1}$) and elite Swedish (14.6 $g\,dl^{-1}$) distance runners. Other endurance athletes also display normal haemoglobin concentrations, despite increased plasma volume levels. During the 1989 World Cross-Country Skiing Championships in Finland, Turner (1996) reported 2% of the male athletes assessed had haemoglobin levels below 14 $g\,dl^{-1}$ and no female competitors had lower than 12 $g\,dl^{-1}$. These findings suggest that haemoglobin concentrations of less that 14 $g\,dl^{-1}$ for male runners and less than $12\,\mathrm{g\,dl^{-1}}$ for female runners may be a sensible threshold for seeking medical advice as a precautionary measure.

Determination of Blood Haematocrit

Haematocrit refers to the relative volume of red blood cells, usually expressed as a percentage of total blood volume. The normal haematocrit ranges between 42–54% for men and 38–46% for women athletes. It should be noted that haematocrit values will be artificially elevated if a runner is assessed when they are in a dehydrated state. Furthermore, as plasma volume changes significantly with changes in posture, it is recommended that subjects sit quietly for 10–20 min before determination of both haemoglobin concentration and haematocrit levels.

Determination of Lung Function

Though not essential, it is probably useful to undergo a test of lung function whilst attending a laboratory-based physiological assessment. Lung function is not normally a determinant of middle or long-distance running performance, but the information obtained can be used as an initial screen for exercise-induced asthma (EIA). This is achieved through comparing lung function at rest to that obtained 5–15 min after a (maximal) $\dot{V}O_{2max}$ test. A decrease of greater than 10–15% in either the peak expiratory flow rate (PEFR) or the volume of air exhaled in the first second of the test (FEV_1), when both are expressed as a percentage of the pre-exercise value is usually indicative of airway narrowing caused by exercise-induced asthma (Morton 1992). This may range from mild (15–25%) to severe (> 50%). It should be emphasised that this will only be an initial screen for EIA and runners are recommended to consult their medical physician if they have any respiratory concerns.

Determination of Maximum Oxygen Uptake ($\dot{V}O_{2max}$)

Maximum oxygen uptake ($\dot{V}O_{2max}$) should be measured directly during a maximal test by collecting and analysing expired air. The maximal test should be performed on a motorised treadmill as lower values (5–10%) are usually reported by runners using cycle ergometers. This is not surprising bearing in mind the specificity of training adaptations discussed in Chapter 5. Expired air is collected either continuously using an on-line gas analysis system (Figure 6.1) or intermittently using the Douglas bag technique (Figure 6.2). Although on-line systems display results immediately, look 'high-tech' and allow analysis of $\dot{V}O_2$ kinetics at the onset of exercise, their validity is sometimes called into question. At present, Douglas bag procedures should be viewed as a 'gold' standard method by which an on-line system should be individually evaluated.

A number of indirect predictive tests have become increasingly popular within the health and fitness industry over the last decade. These tests often use the heart rate response to submaximal exercise to predict $\dot{V}O_{2max}$ but are notoriously unreliable and would be of no benefit to a well-trained runner. The errors associated with predicting $\dot{V}O_{2max}$ using these tests are large; you would be 95% confident that your actual $\dot{V}O_{2max}$ is within $\pm 24\%$ of the value determined by these test. Therefore a $\dot{V}O_{2max}$ of 65 ml kg^{-1} min^{-1} would indicate to the runner that their true $\dot{V}O_{2max}$ was somewhere between 49.5 and 80.6 ml kg^{-1} min^{-1}. This range extends from a sedentary score up to elite 800 m runner potential! Other more promising indirect tests that predict $\dot{V}O_{2max}$ based upon peak running speed attained are discussed later.

The protocol employed for the direct determination of $\dot{V}O_{2max}$ will vary between different laboratories. However, contemporary protocols are usually continuous incremental tests involving increases in speed, gradient or a combination of both. The increments might either be staged

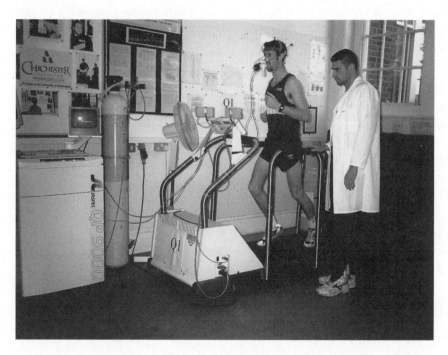

Figure 6.1. On-line gas collection and analysis system

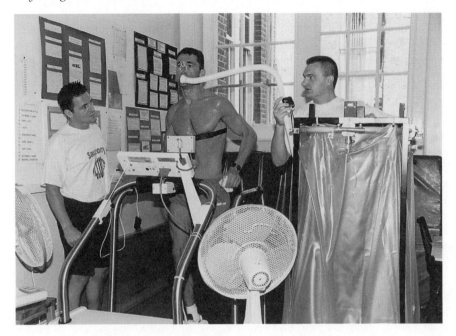

Figure 6.2. Off-line Douglas bag gas collection system

(i.e. step-wise) or ramped (i.e. continually increasing). Nevertheless, there are a number of issues that should be considered when evaluating different procedures. First, the rate of increase in exercise intensity should ensure that the total test duration is approximately 8–12 min in duration. Second, it is important to realise that increasing speed protocols on a flat treadmill usually result in lower $\dot{V}O_{2max}$ values than progressively increasing gradient protocols, by about 4% (Draper, Wood and Fallowfield 1998). This is an important consideration as tests that finish at a steep gradient (10% or more) will produce artificially high $\dot{V}O_{2max}$ values that are not representative of the actual value attained during flat track running. This will in turn lead to an underestimation of the sustainable $\%\dot{V}O_{2max}$ attained during flat track running.

The obvious solution to this problem is to perform all $\dot{V}O_{2max}$ tests on a flat treadmill as the majority of middle and long-distance events are track based. This is not easy for untrained runners who are not familiar with the fast leg speeds needed at near-maximal relative exercise intensities. However most trained runners appear to cope well with the protocol, although safety concerns grow with increasing treadmill speed. This is especially apparent in highly motivated runners, whose concentration and coordination may waiver as they challenge their limits of exhaustion. Furthermore, the running speeds attained near the end of a flat $\dot{V}O_{2max}$ test in highly trained middle-distance runners may exceed the maximum speed of some treadmills. In these circumstances a gradient is often used in order to alleviate these speed concerns.

A possible compromise that has been used successfully in our laboratory over the last few years (Draper, Wood and Fallowfield 1998) has been to increase the gradient at the start of the test by 1% min^{-1} during the first 5 min, and then only increase the speed after this time (by 0.1 km h^{-1} 5 s^{-1}). This has two distinct advantages over the more common constant speed and increasing gradient protocols. First, the final gradient attained is predetermined and can be selected to minimise the protocol-specific increase in $\dot{V}O_{2max}$ associated with steep gradient protocols. Our laboratory has found a 5% gradient to be a good compromise with only a 2% higher $\dot{V}O_{2max}$ being observed in comparison with a flat speed increment protocol (Wood, 1999). In addition, as the final gradient is the same for all subjects, the peak speed achieved at the end of the test can be used for inter-individual comparison, a procedure not possible with variable gradient protocols. Peak treadmill running velocity attained on a $\dot{V}O_{2max}$ test has been shown to be highly related to distance running performance in events ranging from 5 to 90 km (Noakes, Myburgh and Schall 1990, Scott and Houmard 1994) and is a useful additional marker with which to assess changes in training status.

The reliability of measuring oxygen uptake at submaximal and maximal intensities should be within the range of 1.5–3% (Saltin *et al.* 1995a, Jones 1998). Reliability in a test is important, as it will determine the size of the change needed to evaluate whether a runner has improved, stayed the same or has lost fitness. Good measurement reliability will improve the ability to detect the small changes that may occur with training in well-trained distance runners. Individual reliability data on measuring oxygen uptake should be available from all accredited laboratories, and can be used by the runner and coach to confirm the reliability of the system to be used for measuring $\dot{V}O_{2max}$, whether on-line or Douglas bag method.

Typical reported values of $\dot{V}O_{2max}$ for a wide range of well-trained middle and long-distance runners are shown in Table 6.1. Most world class male middle and long-distance runners range from 70–85 ml kg^{-1} min^{-1} and the limited data on female runners suggest values in the range of 63–78 ml kg^{-1} min^{-1}. As a general rule, $\dot{V}O_{2max}$ seems to become more important in males as race distance increases towards 10 km, after which slightly lower values are reported for marathon runners. The limited data on female runners appears to suggest that $\dot{V}O_{2max}$ becomes more important as race distance increases, up to and including the marathon.

Table 6.1. Treadmill $\dot{V}O_{2max}$ for middle and long-distance runners

Athlete/group	Event (M/F)	N	Mean ($1\,min^{-1}$)	Mean ($ml\,kg^{-1}$)	Performance (h:min:s.00)	Reference
Earl Jones	800 m (M)	1	–	72.1	0:01:43.83	Daniels and Daniels (1992)
Swedish elite	800 m (M)	6	4.84	68.8	0:01:49.41	Svedenhag and Sjödin (1984)
Elite	800 m–1500 m (M)	42	4.73	68.9	0:01:48.00–0:03:44.00	Boileau et al. (1982)
Swedish elite	800 m–1500 m (M)	5	4.87	71.9	0:01:49.68–0:03:41.86	Svedenhag and Sjödin (1984)
Elite (mainly USA)	800 m–1500 m (M)	13	5.00	72.5		Daniels and Daniels (1992)
Elite (mainly USA)	800 m–1500 m (F)	8	3.27	63.1		Daniels and Daniels (1992)
Steve Scott	1500 m–1 mile (M)	1	5.85	80.1	0:03:31:96–0:03:49.68	Conley et al. (1984)
Steve Prefontaine	1 mile (M)	1	5.60	84.4	0:03:54.60	Pollock (1977b)
Kip Keino	1500 m–5 km (M)	1		82.0	0:03:34.90–0:13:24.20	Saltin and Astrand (1967)
Swedish elite	1500 m–5 km (M)	6	4.94	75.3*	0:03:44.70–0:13:58.80	Svedenhag and Sjödin (1984)
Peter Koech	3000 m SC (M)	1		85.0*	0:08:10.00	Saltin et al. (1995a)
Paula Ratcliffe	3000 m (F)	1	3.50	66.7	0:08:37:00	Jones et al. (1998)
Elite	3 km–10 km (M)	32	4.96	76.9	0:08:40.00 (SC)–0:29:24.00	Boileau et al. (1982)
Elite (mainly USA)	3 km–10 km (M)	23	4.91	77.4		Daniels and Daniels (1992)
Elite (mainly USA)	3 km–10 km (F)	5	3.51	68.4		Daniels and Daniels (1992)
Swedish elite	5 km–10 km (M)	5	4.92	78.6	0:13:49:90–0:28:57.90	Svedenhag and Sjödin (1984)
Joseph Ngugi	3 km–10 km (M)	1		85.0*		Saltin et al. (1995a)
Henry Rono	10 km (M)	1		84.3	0:27:22.50	Saltin et al. (1995a)
US Olympic trialists	10 km (M)	22	4.86	75.8	0:28:53.40	Morgan and Daniels (1994)
Swedish elite	10 km–42.2 km (M)	5	4.86	73.9	0:29:22.70–2:16:18.00	Svedenhag and Sjödin (1984)
Elite (mainly USA)	42.2 km (M)	9	4.86	74.4		Daniels and Daniels (1992)
Elite (mainly USA)	42.2 km (F)	7	3.62	68.1		Daniels and Daniels (1992)
Derek Clayton	42.2 km (M)	1	5.10	69.7	2:08:33.00	Costill et al. (1971b)
Grete Waitz	42.2 km (F)	1	3.77	73.5	2:25:29.00	Costill (1986)
Joan Benoit[†]	42.2 km (F)	1	–	78.6	2:24:52.00	Daniels and Daniels (1992)

* Estimated values based on related physiological data.
[†] 1984 Olympic marathon champion.
SC Steeplechase

Determination of Running Economy

Chapter 3 defined running economy as the rate of oxygen uptake required to run at a given speed. Therefore at the same race speed, an economical runner will have a lower rate of oxygen uptake in comparison with a less economical runner.

In order to assess running economy, it is first necessary to determine the relationship between running speed and oxygen uptake. This is usually completed on a level motorised treadmill and requires the runner to complete four or five discontinuous exercise stages of increasing running speed, with a 5 min rest between each stage. Both the duration of each stage and the speeds selected for the runs are important factors to consider when determining economy.

The duration of each exercise stage is important because oxygen uptake has to increase at the start of the stage to reach its final stable level or 'steady state'. This takes about 3 min at low exercise intensities ($< 50\%$ $\dot{V}O_{2max}$), with stable values being obtained after this time. At higher exercise intensities above the lactate threshold ($> 70\%$ $\dot{V}O_{2max}$), there is a small but continuing increase in oxygen uptake with a final steady state being reached within 10–20 min. This continued rise in oxygen uptake has been termed the $\dot{V}O_2$ slow component (Gaesser and Poole 1996). Therefore the old concept of oxygen uptake reaching a steady state after 3 min at all exercise intensities needs revision. The duration of the exercise stage at high exercise intensities will influence the rate of oxygen uptake measured, as the oxygen uptake response is time-dependent. From experience in our laboratory, an exercise stage duration of 8 min gives stable oxygen uptake values in well trained runners for the range of exercise intensities usually used in measuring running economy. Regardless of whether on-line or Douglas bag techniques are used, a value of the steady state oxygen uptake should be obtained from the average values measured during the last 2 min of each 8 min stage. The actual range of running speeds employed should span from relatively easy at the slow end (e.g. steady warm-up pace) to just above 10 km race pace at the fast end (Daniels and Daniels 1992). A line on a graph describing the relationship between running speed and the rate of oxygen uptake obtained at these speeds can be derived for an individual runner by linear regression. An equation in the form $y = mX + C$ is obtained, where y is the oxygen uptake ($\text{ml}\,\text{kg}^{-1}\,\text{min}^{-1}$), m is the running speed ($\text{km}\,\text{h}^{-1}$), X is the gradient of the line obtained ($\text{ml}\,\text{kg}^{-1}\,\text{km}^{-1}$) and C is the oxygen uptake value on the graph plotted when speed equals $0\,\text{km}\,\text{h}^{-1}$. If X and C are known, any running speed can be entered into the equation to determine a runner's oxygen cost of running at this speed. For example, Table 6.2 reports the equation for Joseph Ngugi ($y = 3X - 3$), a Kenyan distance runner who has one of the best running economies ever reported (Figure 6.3). Therefore at a treadmill running speed of 16 km h^{-1}, Ngugi requires an oxygen uptake of just 45 ml kg^{-1} min^{-1}.

Running economy can be presented in a number of ways. The rate of oxygen uptake required (ml kg^{-1} min^{-1}) to run at a given speed is the most commonly reported method. Typically this running speed is equivalent to 16 km h^{-1} (approximately 6 min mile^{-1} pace) for well-trained runners. However, Figure 4.11 highlights the fact that although two runners may show similar running economies at a given speed, they may show quite different running economies at a different speed as the slopes of their individual running speed–$\dot{V}O_2$ regression equations are different. This is a particular problem when comparing middle and long-distance runners at 16 km h^{-1}. There is no difference in running economy between middle and long-distance runners when compared at a common slow (marathon pace) speed, but middle-distance runners are considerably more economical than marathon runners when compared at 1500 m speed (Daniels and Daniels 1992). Therefore the chosen speed will determine the conclusion reached when assessing a runner's economy using this method.

A second approach is to report running economy as the millilitres of oxygen used per kilogramme of body weight to run one kilometre (ml kg^{-1} km^{-1}). This can be ascertained using the equation $a = y \times (60/X)$ where a is the oxygen cost (ml kg^{-1} km^{-1}), y is oxygen uptake (ml kg^{-1} min^{-1}) required at running speed X and X is the chosen running speed (km h^{-1}). Applying this approach to the data for Joseph Ngugi (45 ml kg^{-1} min^{-1} at 16 km h^{-1}) would yield an oxygen cost of 169 ml kg^{-1} km^{-1}. This method has received growing support amongst sports scientists as it allows comparison between runners performing at different speeds. However, the oxygen demand of running expressed in this form usually increases with increasing speed, making comparisons only valid when expressed with reference to a specified relative exercise intensity (i.e. %$\dot{V}O_{2max}$). Joseph Ngugi's $\dot{V}O_{2max}$ was estimated at 85 ml kg^{-1} min^{-1} (Table 6.1), his running economy would therefore be expressed as 169 ml kg^{-1} km^{-1} at 53% $\dot{V}O_{2max}$ (i.e. {45 ml kg^{-1} min^{-1} $\div$ 85 ml kg^{-1} min^{-1}} $\times$ 100 = 53% $\dot{V}O_{2max}$). Morgan and Daniels (1994) have reported economy values for 22 elite male distance runners (10 km in 28:53.40) at various relative exercise intensities. Values ranged from 158–195 ml kg^{-1} km^{-1} at 63% $\dot{V}O_{2max}$, 163–197 ml kg^{-1} km^{-1} at 70% $\dot{V}O_{2max}$, 169–200 ml kg^{-1} km^{-1} at 77% $\dot{V}O_{2max}$, and 176–205 ml kg^{-1} km^{-1} at 84% $\dot{V}O_{2max}$. Daniels and Daniels (1992) reported little difference between elite male and elite female distance runners when compared using this method across typical race intensities. Although this approach has the advantage of being able to compare individuals at different

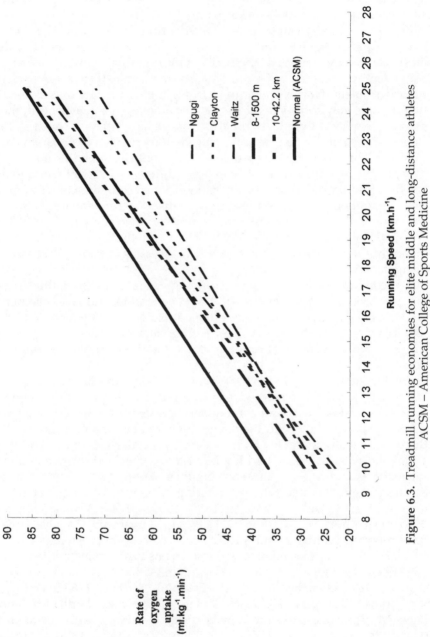

Figure 6.3. Treadmill running economies for elite middle and long-distance athletes
ACSM – American College of Sports Medicine

speeds, or the same relative exercise intensities, it still suffers from the problem that running economy expressed in this way does not always increase with increasing running speed. Daniels and Daniels (1992) reported that despite the majority of runners having an increasing economy as running speed increases, some displayed an equal demand at different speeds, and others a decreasing demand. Once again, the chosen relative exercise intensity used to report running economy may determine the conclusion reached using this method.

Finally, it may be easiest to plot the individual regression line of running speed against oxygen uptake on a graph and compare this in relation to typical lines for other runners. Table 6.2 shows the regression equations for a variety of elite middle and long-distance runners. Any line for any of the athletes or groups shown in Table 6.2 can be plotted using the equations to give a visual impression of running economy across a range of running speeds. It is important to realise that all of the lines shown in Figure 6.3 have been extrapolated to show the theoretical oxygen cost of running at middle-distance race speeds. This extrapolation is based on the assumption that oxygen demand increases linearly with increasing running speed. Also for comparisons to be made between individuals, it is assumed that this energy demand remains constant for the duration of the race if run at a constant speed. Despite the validity of both of these assumptions being challenged at present (Medbo 1996, Bangsbo 1996), there is presently no other satisfactory approach.

Heart rate may be monitored and capillary blood lactate concentrations measured during the submaximal exercise stages of a running economy test. This will allow the heart rate–running speed and blood lactate–running speed relationships to be determined. Chapter 5 discussed the relationship between blood lactate concentration and running perform-ance, where better runners can sustain a higher running speed for a lower blood lactate concentration (Farrell *et al.* 1979, Mader *et al.* 1976, Sjödin and Jacobs 1981). Changes in running performance can be monitored with reference to blood lactate concentrations. A range of approaches have been used to identify an exercise intensity at which blood lactate starts to accumulate. However, the most common practical approach is to determine the running speed equivalent to a reference blood lactate concentration of 2 or 4 mmol$\,$l^{-1} (Sjödin, Jacobs and Svedenhag 1982), where the latter reference concentration is often referred to as OBLA or onset of blood lactate accumulation. Increases or decreases in running performance over time will be evident as higher or lower running speeds sustained at the reference blood lactate concentrations. If the relation-ships between blood lactate concentration, heart rate and running speed are known, it is possible to set levels of training in relation to the stress on the muscle (i.e. peripheral) and the stress on the cardiorespiratory

Table 6.2. Level treadmill running economy equations for middle and long-distance runners

Athlete/group	Event (M/F)	N	$\dot{V}O_2$ (ml kg^{-1} min^{-1}) = speed (km h^{-1})X + C		Performance (h:min:s.00)	Reference
			X (ml kg^{-1} min^{-1} km^{-1} h)	C (ml kg^{-1} min^{-1})		
Swedish elite	800 m (M)	6	3.52	−5.60	0:01:49.41	Svedenhag and Sjödin (1984)
Swedish elite	800–1500 m (M)	5	3.74	−8.30	0:01:49.68–0:03:41.86	Svedenhag and Sjödin (1984)
Elite (mainly USA)	800 m–1500 m (M)	8	3.42	−5.86		Daniels and Daniels (1992)
Elite (mainly USA)	800 m–1500 m (F)	8	3.48	−4.44		Daniels and Daniels (1992)
Steve Scott	1500 m–1 mile (M)	1	3.33	−7.70	0:03:31:96–0:03:49.68	Conley et al. (1984)
Swedish elite	1500 m–5 km (M)	6	3.80	−9.80	0:03:44.70–0:13:58.80	Svedenhag and Sjödin (1984)
Joseph Ngugi	3 km–10 km (M)	1	3.00	−3.00		Saltin et al. (1995a)
Swedish elite	5 km–10 km (M)	5	4.30	−19.90	0:13:49:90–0:28:57.90	Svedenhag and Sjödin (1984)
US Olympic trialists	10 km (M)	22	4.20	−20.04	0:28:53.40	Morgan and Daniels (1994)
Trained runners	10 km (M)	12	3.48	−5.67	0:32:06	Conley and Krahenbuhl (1980)
Swedish elite	10 km–42.2 km (M)	5	3.90	−12.20	0:29:22.70–2:16:18.00	Svedenhag and Sjödin (1984)
Elite (mainly USA)	10 km–42.2 km (M)	8	4.23	−20.99		Daniels and Daniels (1992)
Elite (mainly USA)	10 km–42.2 km (F)	8	4.05	−13.54*		Daniels and Daniels (1992)
Derek Clayton	42.2 km (M)	1	3.21	−4.64	2:08:33.00	Costill et al. (1971b)
Grete Waitz	42.2 km (F)	1	4.01	−17.11	2:25:29.00	Costill (1986)

* Recalculated from Daniels and Daniels (1992) as reported value does not fit the data shown in their Figure 5.

system (i.e. central). This has been discussed in greater detail in Chapter 5 (Technical Box 5.1). When running speed is reported at a fixed blood lactate concentration, the measure is sensitive to changes in $\dot{V}O_{2max}$, running economy and sustainable $\%\dot{V}O_{2max}$, and is therefore highly responsive to changes in training status.

However, there are a number of factors that may influence the interpretation of the blood lactate–running speed relationship. For example, a runner who attends an assessment in the laboratory in an fatigued, over-reached, or overtrained state (Chapter 5) would exhibit an artificially lowered blood lactate concentration at a given running speed. This results in a higher running speed for a reference blood lactate concentration. Low blood lactate concentrations might reflect depleted muscle glycogen stores due to inadequate recovery and/or a diet that fails to replace the runner's carbohydrate stores (Chapter 8), rather than a training response *per se*. Adequate pre-assessment standardisation for the runner prior to performing any activity, in terms of diet and rest, should minimise these problems.

Determination of Sustainable Percentage of $\dot{V}O_{2max}$ ($\%\dot{V}O_{2max}$)

A runner's sustainable $\%\dot{V}O_{2max}$ can be described as the average percentage of $\dot{V}O_{2max}$ a runner can sustain for a prescribed event. This percentage will decrease as race distance, and hence duration, increases. Therefore the importance of sustaining a relatively high percentage of $\dot{V}O_{2max}$ increases with race distance, especially in marathon running.

There are two possible approaches for determining the $\%\dot{V}O_{2max}$ sustained during distance running. The most direct method is to measure oxygen uptake throughout the entire event (Spencer, Gastin and Payne 1996) or over selected time periods during the event (Maron *et al.* 1976, Ramsbottom *et al.* 1992). This may be an actual race or simulated treadmill time trial, although the latter approach is by far the most common for practical reasons (i.e. the runner is stationary). The average oxygen uptake measured over the duration of the event can then be expressed as a percentage of $\dot{V}O_{2max}$. It is important to remember that as the duration of the distance races decreases to 1500 m and below, this average $\%\dot{V}O_{2max}$ will progressively underestimate the final $\%\dot{V}O_{2max}$ sustained over the latter part of the race, due to the increasing percentage of the total race time over which the rate of oxygen uptake is increasing. Hence, the average $\%\dot{V}O_{2max}$ reported by Spencer, Gastin and Payne (1996) in a simulated 800 m run was approximately 81% $\dot{V}O_{2max}$. However, the final $\%\dot{V}O_{2max}$ maintained over the latter half of this run was 94% $\dot{V}O_{2max}$. Therefore it is important to discriminate between the average $\%\dot{V}O_{2max}$

sustained over the duration of a race and the final $\%\dot{V}O_{2max}$ attained over the final part of the race for middle-distance events.

The second, and perhaps the most widely adopted approach would be to estimate $\%\dot{V}O_{2max}$ sustained from an actual race performance. This would require a runner to determine their regression equation describing the relationship between running speed and oxygen uptake, described previously for assessing running economy. From a runner's race time for a given event, it is possible to calculate the average race speed sustained and use their regression equation to determine the estimated $\dot{V}O_2$ demand to run at this speed. This estimated $\dot{V}O_2$ demand can then be expressed as a percentage of $\dot{V}O_{2max}$ to give the estimated $\%\dot{V}O_{2max}$ sustained.

It important to note that this is a theoretical oxygen demand and this demand is likely to be above 100% $\dot{V}O_{2max}$ in middle-distance events due to the significant contribution from anaerobic metabolism to total energy production in these shorter events (Chapter 3). If the quantification of the actual aerobic contribution to these middle-distance events is required, direct measurement of oxygen uptake in a laboratory will need to be made. The difference between the estimated $\dot{V}O_2$ demand and the actual $\dot{V}O_2$ supply in 5 and 10 km races will be smaller, but not insignificant, especially in those runners with a high anaerobic capacity (Figure 4.9). This difference will be negligible in half-marathon and marathon races.

An additional problem with this second approach is that the estimated $\dot{V}O_2$ demand will underestimate the actual $\dot{V}O_2$ supply if an outdoor race time is used with a regression equation derived from a treadmill run. This is due to the treadmill regression equation ignoring the additional oxygen cost of overcoming air resistance. This underestimation will be greater as the average race speed increases, and hence the oxygen cost of overcoming air resistance increases. An estimation of the actual $\%\dot{V}O_{2max}$ sustained can be achieved by correcting the estimated $\dot{V}O_2$ demand, using the equation proposed by di Prampero (1986). The effect of correcting $\%\dot{V}O_{2max}$ for air resistance during a marathon race is shown in Figure 6.4 using data derived from Maughan and Leiper (1983). For a 2:10:00 marathon runner, this represents a change from ~80 to 86% $\dot{V}O_{2max}$. Once again it is important to note that this difference will be affected by racing tactics such as drafting, change in course terrain and prevailing environmental conditions. Finally, the $\%\dot{V}O_{2max}$ sustained decreases as race duration increases (Davies and Thompson 1979, Maughan and Leiper 1983) and so comparisons between individuals should only be made with similar race times, or an estimation made to correct for the likely effect of increasing race duration. Values for a variety of middle and long-distance runners are shown in Table 6.3.

In summary, middle-distance and 5 km runners will need to have oxygen uptake directly measured during a simulated race to derive useful information on the $\%\dot{V}O_{2max}$ attained or sustained during the run. If performed using an on-line analysis system, information of $\dot{V}O_2$ kinetics will also be available and can be used to assess training progress. Ten kilometre, half-marathon and marathon runners will be able to use race times and running economy data to estimate their $\%\dot{V}O_{2max}$ sustained during the race, especially on flat courses on calm days once corrected for air resistance.

Determination of Anaerobic Capacity

In Chapter 3 the relative importance of anaerobic capacity was discussed as a determinant of middle-distance running performance. There is a great deal of controversy surrounding its measurement (Bangsbo 1996, Medbo 1996), with the maximal accumulated oxygen deficit (MAOD) approach being the most promising method at present despite its theoretical limitations (Green and Dawson 1993). The MAOD procedure requires the runner to perform a supramaximal ($> \dot{V}O_{2max}$) constant exercise bout to exhaustion. This speed is determined by extending their

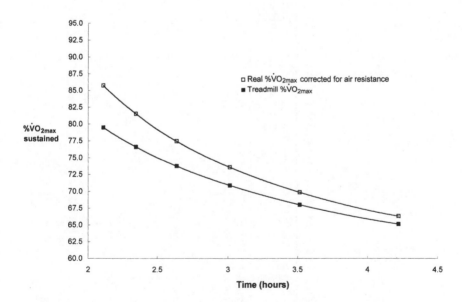

Figure 6.4. $\%\dot{V}O_{2max}$ sustained as a function of marathon time with and without a correction for air resistance (calculated from data presented by Maughan and Leiper 1983)

Table 6.3. Estimated treadmill and measured sustained $\%\dot{V}O_{2max}$ values reported for middle and long-distance runners

Athlete/group	Event (M/F)	N	Mean (range) estimated $\%\dot{V}O_{2max}$	Mean (range) estimated* $\%\dot{V}O_{2max}$	Measured $\%\dot{V}O_{2max}$	Performance (h:min:s.00)	Reference
Swedish elite	800 m (M)	6	127	143		0:01:49.41	Svedenhag and Sjödin (1984)
Swedish elite	1500 m (M)	5	115	128		0:03:41.86	Svedenhag and Sjödin (1984)
Elite Kenyans	3000 m (SC)				98		Saltin et al. (1995a)
P.E. students	5 km (M)	59	87	91		0:19:46.20	Ramsbottom, Nute and Williams (1987)
P.E. students	5 km (F)	44	88	89		0:24:26.40	Ramsbottom, Nute and Williams (1987)
Recreational	5 km (M)	8			90	0:17:40.80	Ramsbottom et al. (1992)
Recreational	5 km (F)	8			88	0:18:46.20	Ramsbottom et al. (1992)
Runners	5 km (M)	13	94 (89–100)	99		0:15:49.20	Davies and Thompson (1979)
Swedish elite	5 km (M)	5	93	102		0:13:49.90	Svedenhag and Sjödin (1984)
Elite Kenyans	5 km		98				Saltin et al. (1995a)
Runners	10 km (M)	12	83	89		0:32:06.00	Morgan et al. (1989)
Swedish elite	10 km (M)	5	88	96		0:28:57.90	Svedenhag and Sjödin (1984)
Elite Kenyans	10 km				95		Saltin et al. (1995a)
Runners	10 km (M)	4	86 (75–95)			0:37:06.00	Scrimgeour et al. (1986)
Elite runners	16 km (M)		86 (82–90)	93 (90–97)		0:49:24.00	Costill, Thomason and Roberts (1973)

Elite runners	16 km (M)	4	88 (83–90)	94 (89–97)	0:53:04.00	Costill, Thomason and Roberts (1973)
Elite runners	16 km (M)	4	87 (86–92)	92 (86–98)	0:58:12.00	Costill, Thomason and Roberts (1973)
Elite runners	16 km (M)	4	84 (81–91)	88 (85–95)	1:04:42.00	Costill, Thomason and Roberts (1973)
Runners	21.1 km (M)	1	81 (68–91)		1:23:00.00	Scrimgeour et al. (1986)
Derek Clayton	42.2 km (M)		86	91	2:08:33.00	Costill et al. (1971b)
Swedish elite	42.2 km (M)	5	82	87	2:16:18.00	Svedenhag and Sjödin (1984)
Distance	42.2 km	12	80 (73–84)	87	2:21:00.00	Sjödin and Svedenhag (1985)
Distance	42.2 km	16	80 (74–84)	86	2:37:00.00	Sjödin and Svedenhag (1985)
Distance	42.2 km	7	71 (59–79)	74	3:24:00.00	Sjödin and Svedenhag (1985)
Marathoners	42.2 km (M)	5	74 (58–76)	78	2:34:42.00	Maughan and Leiper (1983)
Marathoners	42.2 km (F)	3	76 (57–79)	80	3:04:20.00	Maughan and Leiper (1983)
Marathon	42.2 km (M)	2		79	2:38:00.00	Maron et al. (1976)
Runners	42.2 km (M)	13	82 (76–87)	85	2:30:06.00	Davies and Thompson (1979)
Runners	42.2 km (M)	12	67 (53–76)	70	5:57:39.00	Davies and Thompson (1979)
Runners	42.2 km (F)	9	79 (68–87)	82	3:09:36.00	Davies and Thompson (1979)
Runners	42.2 km (M)		75 (58–87)		2:56:30.00	Scrimgeour et al. (1986)
Runners	56 km (M)		67 (43–85)		4:23:54.00	Scrimgeour et al. (1986)
Runners	90 km (M)		57 (27–70)		7:56:36.00	Scrimgeour et al. (1986)

* Estimated treadmill value corrected for air resistance.

As the races become shorter, the contribution from anaerobic metabolism will increase and the difference between the estimated and measured $\%\dot{V}O_{2max}$ will increase.

individual running speed $-\dot{V}O_2$ regression line up to the required $\dot{V}O_2$ demand (%$\dot{V}O_{2max}$). Through continuous collection of expired air, the actual $\dot{V}O_2$ supply can be measured. You will recall from Chapter 3 that the difference between the $\dot{V}O_2$ demand and the $\dot{V}O_2$ supply represents the anaerobic contribution to energy production, which can be calculated in terms of an equivalent oxygen cost. It is assumed that as the supramaximal exercise bout lasts more than two minutes and is an exhaustive exercise bout, the runner will have depleted their anaerobic capacity (Chapter 3). This test therefore estimates the anaerobic capacity in terms of the calculated accumulated oxygen deficit ($\dot{V}O_2$ demand $-\dot{V}O_2$ supply) and considers the deficit maximum, as the anaerobic capacity should have been exhausted at the end of the test. This concept is illustrated in Figure 3.5.

Criticism of the MAOD test has focused on the two previously mentioned assumptions relating to extrapolating the $-\dot{V}O_2$ running speed relationship. That is, it assumes that the relationship remains linear (especially at supramaximal speeds) and that the $\dot{V}O_2$ demand remains constant as long as the running speed remains the same. However, the MAOD has been shown to be the same under conditions of altered oxygen availability and is unaffected by the length of the exercise bout as long as it exceeds two minutes (Medbo *et al.* 1988). As there is no other acceptable approach to assessing anaerobic capacity, the MAOD has been used to quantify the limited data available on middle and long-distance runners in Table 6.4. Although slightly different methodologies have been used in Table 6.4, all exhaustive runs were over two minutes in duration, as shorter periods may be too brief to deplete fully the anaerobic capacity (Medbo *et al.* 1988).

There are no clear method guidelines as to the most effective approach for assessing MAOD at present, with virtually all studies using a modification of the original Medbo *et al.* (1988) method. However, some points are worthy of consideration. First, the number of data points used to determine the individual running speed $-\dot{V}O_2$ regression should be as large as possible. Small differences in the gradient of this line could have a large influence on the final estimated $\dot{V}O_2$ demand, especially at high exercise intensities. Although 120% $\dot{V}O_{2max}$ is commonly used to determine the speed for the supramaximal exercise bout, 105% $\dot{V}O_{2max}$ would reduce the extrapolation errors in calculating the $\dot{V}O_2$ demand. This would also ensure that the duration of the exercise bout would be increased from the usual 2–4 min to 4–10 min, eliminating the chances of runners not exhausting their anaerobic capacity during the run. It would also reduce the required treadmill speed needed to elicit 105% $\dot{V}O_{2max}$, allowing many club level runners to perform the test on a flat treadmill. The regression data will then also be useful for assessing running

Table 6.4. Maximum accumulated oxygen deficits during treadmill running (> 2 min) for middle and long-distance runners

Athlete/group	Event (M/F)	N	Mean range (ml kg^{-1})	Performance (min:s.00)	Reference
Untrained		4	62 (45–78)		Medbo et al. (1988)
Benson Koech	800 m (M)	1	> 100	01:43.00	Saltin et al. (1995a)
Elite Kenyans	800–5 km (M)	5	77*	01:47.00–13:21.00	Svedenhag et al. (1991)
European	1500 m	1	860	3:35.00	Bangsbo, Michalsik and Peterson (1993)
Middle distance		3	75 (73–78)		Medbo et al. (1988)
Sprint trained		1	82		Medbo et al. (1988)
Endurance trained	3000 m +	4	56		Scott et al. (1991)
Middle distance	800 m –1500 m	5	74		Scott et al. (1991)
Sprint trained	200 m –400 m	3	78		Scott et al. (1991)
Endurance trained		3	58		Green (1990)
Good distance runners	800 m –10 km	14	52 (27–86)	01:49.00–28:40.00	Bangsbo, Michalsik and Peterson (1993)

* Six days after returning from a two-week training camp at 2000 m.

economy. At higher exercise intensities, all regressions and supramaximal tests have to be performed up an inclined treadmill, due to the limitations of the top speed of most motorised treadmills. Finally, the runners performing the test should be given maximum verbal encouragement as the exhaustive test is mentally challenging.

PERFORMANCE TESTS FOR PREDICTING PHYSIOLOGICAL VARIABLES

There are a limited number of field-based tests, particularly for the determination of $\dot{V}O_{2max}$, which might be adapted for the assessment of middle and long-distance running performance. The Multi-stage Shuttle Running Test (MSRT) was designed to assess peak running speed and predict $\dot{V}O_{2max}$ in athletes (Ramsbottom, Brewer and Williams 1988). The MSRT is a step-incremental test that requires runners to perform 20 m shuttle runs, where the required running speed is increased by 0.14 m s^{-1} each minute (or level). The required running speed is dictated to the runner by an audio cue and the increase in running speed at the end of each level is indicated by a verbal cue. The test is widely used by many sporting organisations and has been shown to predict $\dot{V}O_{2max}$ to within $\pm 3.5 \text{ ml kg}^{-1} \text{ min}^{-1}$. However, the verbal cues on the cassette allow athletes to goal set, so the final score may not simply reflect their physiological status. In order to negate the effects of goal setting, Wilkinson, Fallowfield and Myers (1999) have developed a modified shuttle running test which eliminates the need for verbal cues. Similar to the MSRT, $\dot{V}O_{2max}$ can be predicted from the modified test. Both shuttle-run tests principally measure peak running speed, and as such will be more sensitive to training adaptations than a direct measure of $\dot{V}O_{2max}$. This is because peak running speed is influenced by a combination of $\dot{V}O_{2max}$, running economy and anaerobic capacity (Billat and Koralsztein 1996). Thus, shuttle-run tests can provide the runner and coach with an easily accessible and sensitive method of monitoring change in training status.

KEY POINTS

- In the United Kingdom, the British Association of Sport and Exercise Sciences awards accreditation to both laboratories and personnel who have demonstrated that they can offer a high-quality professional service for the physiological assessment of athletes.
- Careful physical and nutritional preparation should precede any form

of physiological assessment, to ensure that the results reflect the runner's true capabilities and are not influenced by recent racing, training, or dietary practices.

- The determination of height, weight, blood haemoglobin concentration, haematocrit and resting lung function (repeated 5–15 min after maximal exercise) are useful preliminary measures in a physiological assessment programme.
- Oxygen uptake is a routine measure in most exercise laboratories and is determined by collecting expired air into Douglas bags for subsequent analysis or processed in real-time by on-line gas analysers.
- Maximal oxygen uptake should be determined during incremental treadmill running on a flat or moderately inclined grade (5%), to avoid the unrealistically high values obtained with the classical increasing gradient protocols.
- Running economy is usually determined by completing four or five discontinuous exercise stages of 8 min duration with a 5 min rest between each stage. Despite a number of different approaches that can be used to express running economy, the simplest and most informative would be to plot the regression line relating running speed and the rate of oxygen uptake on a graph (Figure 6.3).
- If blood lactate concentration is determined during the running economy test, the speed at an appropriate lactate threshold can be derived. Although this can be a useful measure for monitoring changes in performance or setting training intensities remember it is not a component of middle and long-distance running performance as it stands (see Figures 3.14 and 4.14).
- The $\%\dot{V}O_{2max}$ attained/sustained during middle distance and 5 km races will need to be determined directly during a simulation. For 10 km races and above, the $\%\dot{V}O_{2max}$ sustained may be estimated from race speed and running economy, especially when performed on flat courses on calm days, once corrected for air resistance.
- Controversy surrounds the estimation of anaerobic capacity, but the only practical solution at present is to calculate the maximal accumulated oxygen deficit after performing a constant speed run to exhaustion at somewhere between 105–120% $\dot{V}O_{2max}$.
- The only field tests available to the runner and coach at present that estimate $\dot{V}O_{2max}$ with any degree of accuracy are those based on multistage shuttle running, using peak running speed to estimate $\dot{V}O_{2max}$.

Chapter 7

Running and Tissue Damage

Robert B. Child

INTRODUCTION

The physiological adaptations to training, which are associated with improved middle and long-distance running performance, have been discussed in Chapter 5. Despite these adaptations, which help the body to cope with the challenge of exercise, there is increasing recognition that the stresses imposed by training and competition can also be harmful. In a study monitoring 62 distance runners over an 18 to 20 month period, 85% of the athletes sustained at least one training related injury (Bovens *et al.* 1989). Anecdotal reports suggest elite runners have a similar susceptibility to injury. In middle and long-distance events at most of the recent World Championship and Olympic Games, at least one potential medalist has not competed or has retired in the preliminary rounds of competition as a consequence of injury. Notable cases at the 1996 Olympic Games include Kelly Holmes (800 m) and Haile Gebrselassie (5000 and 10 000 m). This chapter outlines mechanisms of cellular and tissue damage associated with middle and long-distance running, and examines some of the practical interventions which may help in optimising adaptation, minimising injury and enhancing performance.

Revisiting the nature of the training stimulus may provide some clues to help explain the relatively high incidence of injury in runners supposedly in peak condition. Training for middle and long-distance running is based upon the principle of overload. In overloading the physiological systems which underpin running performance, the body's equilibrium is disturbed, right down to the cellular level. This triggers a host of adaptive responses which can produce the desired training effects. Paradoxically, the training programmes undertaken by runners, though ultimately resulting in adaptation, initially cause tissue injury. For example, the mitochondria providing aerobic energy to fuel muscle contraction may initially be damaged by endurance training (Davies *et al.* 1982). Thus, the nature of the training stimulus is such that tissue injuries will be present even in well-conditioned runners (Hikida *et al.* 1983, Warhol *et al.* 1985, Kuipers *et al.* 1989).

To allow adaptation, a balance must be found between applying the training stimulus and allowing sufficient time for tissue to repair. Despite the apparent simplicity of this concept, problems arise in identifying the optimal frequency and intensity of effort to maximise training benefits (Rowbottom, Keast and Morton 1998), whilst also preventing the accumulation of excessive tissue damage. This problem is further complicated by the different rates of tissue repair, resulting in comparatively minor injuries taking several days or even weeks to fully recover (Medoff 1987, Bovens *et al.* 1989, Chilibeck, Sale and Webber 1995).

During periods of high-volume training, the processes of tissue repair may not take place quickly enough to maintain optimal tissue functioning. As a result, many runners may have a relatively high proportion of tissues in a damaged state. These runners are likely to under-perform during training and competition, or may not even be able to perform at all. The former condition is potentially dangerous, as a highly motivated athlete may push themselves to train, further aggravating acute minor damage into a major chronic injury.

DEFINING TISSUE INJURY

Training for middle and long-distance running imposes considerable metabolic, biomechanical and cardiorespiratory demands on the athlete (Sjödin and Svedenhag 1985). There is now increasing evidence to link these physiological demands with the incidence of tissue injuries. However, there is tremendous diversity in the nature and aetiology of injury resulting from these training demands. Runners and coaches typically relate the term *injury* to gross structural failures such as tears or ruptures in muscle, tendons and ligaments, and fractures in bone. These, whilst serious, are comparatively rare. In contrast, injuries at the opposite end of the continuum, involving damage to cell membranes or biochemical changes within muscle fibres are far more common. Despite the less obvious nature of these injuries, the resulting damage may be equally debilitating for the runner in terms of maintaining running performance.

Thus, tissue injury refers to a disruption of the normal structure and/or functioning of any part of the body. There are many mechanisms through which tissue might become injured during middle and long-distance running. However, ischaemia, metabolic stress, hyperthermia and high mechanical loadings are probably the most damaging.

ISCHAEMIC INJURY

Ischaemia refers to a local and temporary deficiency in blood supply to tissues. Exercise is associated with circulatory changes, which prioritise blood flow to active muscles (providing oxygen and nutrients, whilst removing unwanted metabolites and heat) and skin (to facilitate the dissipation of heat). Increased circulation to muscle and skin can deprive the gut, liver and kidneys of blood over prolonged periods, making these tissues susceptible to ischaemic injury. The restoration of a normal blood supply following ischaemia is associated with increased formation of reactive chemicals called *free radicals* (McCord 1985, Gauduel, Mendsche and Duvellroy 1989). The term free radical refers to a chemical group that has one or more unpaired electrons in the outer orbit of the molecule (Halliwell and Chirico 1993). These potentially destructive radicals can be formed at increased rates in several tissues following exercise. Antioxidants are compounds which have the capacity to neutralise free radicals, thereby preventing their harmful effects. However, if the rate of free radical production exceeds the antioxidant defences of a tissue, oxidative damage will occur resulting in damage to cell membranes and impaired muscle function.

HYPERTHERMIA

Even well-trained runners are rarely able to convert more than 25% of the available metabolic energy into mechanical work. The majority of the remaining energy is lost in the form of heat. The running speeds sustained by elite marathon runners requires nearly 1000 W of heat energy to be dissipated from the body. The resulting thermal challenge is equivalent to keeping the internal temperature of a small cupboard below 41 °C when heated by a single bar electric fire! It is therefore not surprising that runners have difficulty in maintaining a constant body temperature and that heat illness following long-distance races is common.

The most effective method of heat dissipation for the runner is through the evaporation of sweat from the skin's surface (Chapter 9). During intense exercise (especially in warm environments), where high rates of fluid loss may result in dehydration, the ability to maintain a stable core temperature would become compromised. When fluid loss exceeds approximately 3% body weight (e.g. 2.0 l for a runner weighing 65 kg) core temperature rises rapidly, even in temperate conditions of less than 17 °C (Wyndham and Strydom 1969). In the later stages of a long-distance event, core temperature may exceed 40–41 °C (Costill 1972, Maron, Wagner and Horvath 1977, Pugh, Corbett and Johnson 1967). Such high core temperatures do not always lead to impaired performance in trained runners during the event (Maron, Wagner and Horvath 1977), but may contribute to ischaemic tissue damage following exercise.

GUT INJURY

The gut (stomach, intestines and colon) has been reported to be the most common site of exercise-related medical problems following long-distance running (Halvorsen and Ritland 1992). The most frequently reported symptoms include diarrhoea, vomiting and the presence of blood in faeces (McMahon *et al*. 1984, McCabe *et al*. 1986, Noakes 1991, Fisher *et al*. 1986). The severity of injury experienced by some runners is illustrated by the statement by Derek Clayton after setting the world marathon record in 1967:

> *Two hours later the elation had worn off; I was urinating large dots of blood and was vomiting black mucus and had a lot of black diarrhoea. I don't think too many people can understand what I went through for the next 48 hours* (Runners World, May 1979, p72)

Loss of blood from the gastrointestinal tract is of particular concern as it demonstrates that the gut wall has been damaged, thereby allowing digestive bacteria (normally retained within the gastrointestinal tract) to enter the blood. This can cause secondary problems including toxic shock, sepsis, inflammation (Kraft *et al*. 1992) and liver damage (Kasravi *et al*. 1996). Gut injury could therefore ultimately result in damage to other organs by exposing them to toxic agents. The severity of such injury may be further increased by concurrent ischaemic damage to the liver and kidneys, facilitating the entry of blood borne toxins.

There may be both metabolic and mechanical components to exercise-induced gut injury. During intense exercise, blood flow to some regions of the gut is reduced by 50–80% (Qamer and Read 1987). These circulatory changes may be sufficient to produce ischaemic gut injury (Fisher *et al*. 1986). Such damage could contribute to lesions in the upper digestive tract following long-distance running (Gaudin, Zerath and Guezennec 1990).

Exercise-induced dehydration increases both the severity and duration of ischaemia, and has been associated with increases in gut complaints in athletes (Rehrer *et al.* 1990). The higher frequency of gastrointestinal problems reported during running in comparison with other endurance sports (Halvorsen and Ritland 1992) might reflect the additional mechanical loading on the musculoskeletal system. The repetitive jarring of the intestine, and its contents, may exacerbate problems arising from ischaemia and/or hyperthermia (Halvorsen and Ritland 1992).

MECHANICAL DAMAGE

The body weight of the runner, the biomechanics of foot motion, running shoe design, and the use of orthotics, all contribute to the mechanical loadings experienced by the body during running. This section addresses the effects of forces applied through the lower extremity of the body on tissue damage at the cellular level.

The characteristics of mechanical loadings which result in structural failure have been studied extensively by engineers. Similar techniques have been applied to the study of mechanical damage in biological structures such as bone, connective tissue and skeletal muscle. As a consequence, much of the terminology used to describe the manner in which loadings are applied to biological tissues are derived from those used in mechanical engineering. Two factors which appear to be important for the initiation of mechanical damage in tissue are the force applied per unit cross-sectional area (i.e. mechanical stress) and the change in length of a structure relative to its resting length (i.e. strain). The magnitude of mechanical stress and strain experienced during running appears to be directly related to the damage produced in bone and soft tissues (muscle, tendons, fascia, ligaments).

Mechanical loadings during running are applied to the musculoskeletal system through impact forces between the foot and the ground. On level ground (e.g. track running), these forces can be three to four times greater than a runner's body weight. However, during downhill running the forces are even greater. This is due to the increase in time over which the force of gravity is acting upon the body, and rises in proportion to the steepness of the slope.

As a consequence of high impact forces acting through the foot, most mechanically induced running injuries occur in the lower extremity. The connective tissues of ligaments, tendons and cartilage in these areas, and the bone matrix of the lower limbs, are particularly susceptible to mechanical damage. Injury can also affect the locomotory muscles of the lower limbs, especially those muscles which contract eccentrically to absorb foot strike impact forces. These muscles include the *tibialis anterior* (which dorsiflects the foot) and *quadriceps* (which produces extension at the knee joint). The compressive forces applied during the ground contact phase of the running action may also contribute to rupture of red blood cells in the capillaries and arterioles of the foot (Miller, Pale and Burgess 1988, Smith 1995). The mechanical trauma to tissue resulting from ground impact forces can be ascribed to simple overload, muscle fatigue reducing shock absorbence, hard and/or irregular running surfaces and the repeated application of low stresses over long periods of time (Frankel 1978).

SOFT TISSUE INJURY

Although a pulled or torn muscle is a frequently diagnosed soft tissue injury, very little is known about the structural changes which occur at the site of injury. Muscle is composed of cellular contractile units (muscle fibres) which facilitate the application of force through the skeleton, thereby producing or resisting movement. These individual fibres are bonded together by a complex net-like lattice, which is made up of the protein *collagen* (Figure 7.1). This lattice fuses into parallel strands of collagen to form a tendon, which is then inserted into bone to provide anchorage for the muscle. Tendons may contribute to shock absorption during foot strike, providing some degree of protection to the muscle fibres.

Ligaments are made up of fibrous connective tissue, with each end attached to a bone. Their role is to resist abnormal or unwanted joint motion, thereby providing stability to the musculoskeletal system. Liga-

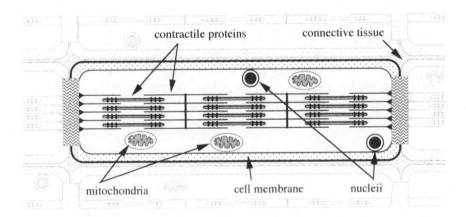

Figure 7.1. Illustration of a longitudinal section through a skeletal muscle showing a single muscle fibre in relation to adjacent muscle fibres

ments are primarily comprised of collagen. Rather than arranging the collagen strands linearly (as in a tendon), in ligaments they are woven into a matrix to provide greater stretch at the expense of stiffness or rigidity. This elastic property of ligaments is further enhanced by the presence of the protein *elastin*. The orientation of fibres, and the number of crosslinks between fibres, determines the biomechanical properties of a tissue. For example, the linear alignment of collagen fibres in the *Achilles tendon* provides greater stiffness (for a given cross-sectional area), than the matrix arrangement of collagen fibres in the *anterior cruciate* ligament which is more elastic.

The mechanics of the collagen fibre determine whether a given mechanical stress will result in injury. Collagen fibres might be likened simplistically to a spring. A spring will extend and return to its natural length under low to moderate levels of applied force, and the same is true of collagen fibres. However, if the applied force exceeds the elastic limits of a spring, it will no longer return to its natural length and will remain permanently deformed. Similarly, collagen fibres extended beyond their yield point will fail (Noyes *et al.* 1974) and such damage represents the early stages of injury to connective tissue. Further increases in the applied force beyond this yield point will result in rupture of the tissue (Noyes, DeLucas and Torvik 1974, Noyes *et al.* 1974). However, the force necessary to rupture the tissue is less than that applied at the yield point (Noyes, DeLucas and Torvik 1974, Noyes *et al.* 1974), as initial tearing (at the yield point) reduces the tissue's maximum load-bearing capabilities. From a practical perspective, this means that the application of moderate forces to injured or structurally weakened tissues may result in much greater damage than could be predicted from the applied force.

In addition to fibre structure and orientation, the rate and frequency of tissue loading also influences the nature of injury. If an excessive load is slowly applied to the *anterior cruciate* ligament, failure occurs at the point where the ligament attaches to the bone. In contrast, rapid loading of a tissue is more likely to result in interstitial tearing, or rupture within the tissue (Noyes, DeLucas and Torvik 1974). Another factor determining a runner's susceptibility to injury is their training history. Habitual physical conditioning typically develops the absolute strength of soft tissue, thereby improving its ability to resist excessive external forces. However, it may take up to six months of training to produce the adaptations which improve resistance to the damage caused by high forces (Noyes *et al.* 1974, Tipton *et al.* 1975). In contrast, as little as two weeks of inactivity can result in significant reductions in the resistive qualities of fibres in muscle and connective tissue (Amiel *et al.* 1983). This means that even brief periods of disuse will leave these tissues less able to resist mechanical loadings and therefore more prone to injury (Noyes *et al.* 1974).

Soft tissue injury can result in delayed onset muscle soreness (DOMS), which usually peaks two to three days after particularly strenuous training or downhill running. Soreness appears to be a symptom of inflammatory processes at the site of damage (Hikida *et al.* 1983), involving the accumulation of *neutrophils* (white blood cells involved in killing bacteria and destroying tissue) and *macrophages* (scavenger cells also involved in destroying bacteria and breaking down damaged tissue). Inflammation of muscle tissue can be evident as little as an hour after damaging exercise (Fielding *et al.* 1993) and may last for longer than a week (Child *et al.* 1999).

Hydrocortisone (cortisol) is a hormone that is released from the adrenal glands during exercise, which has a strong anti-inflammatory effect. It suppresses both macrophage invasion and the accumulation of *fibroblasts*, the cells responsible for the generation of new collagen fibres at the site of injury. As hydrocortisone production is elevated during periods of intense training, connective tissue repair may be reduced at a time when the possibility of exercise-induced connective tissue injury is increased. This potentially unfavourable balance between tissue damage and tissue repair may be a contributing factor to the high incidence of connective tissue injuries reported during intense periods of training and competition.

Inflammation within a tendon is symptomatic of the commonly diagnosed injury, tendonitis. This injury usually results from repeated loading of a tendon beyond its yield point. Thus, inflammation may be more a response to, rather than a cause of, soft tissue injury (Medoff 1987). Inflamed tissues may be more susceptible to mechanically induced injury, as like mechanically damaged tissues their load-bearing capabilities may be compromised. This probably arises from the enzymatic degradation of damaged (and possibly undamaged) tissue and the synthesis of new connective tissue. Although connective tissue can be synthesised rapidly, in its immature state it has comparatively few cross links, or fibres aligned to cope with applied forces. Structural maturation, which increases the strength of connective tissue, can take several months (Medoff 1987); therefore a rehabilitating runner must be careful not to aggravate sites of previous damage. Too much running ... too soon ... in the recovery programme, may result in renewed and potentially more serious re-injury.

BONE INJURY

Bone provides the attachment sites for tendons, which in turn will allow skeletal muscle to apply force and produce limb movement. Bone has a dynamic structure which is constantly undergoing remodelling. This occurs through the processes of bone breakdown (where *osteoclast* cells destroy old bone cells and remove calcium) and bone formation (where *osteoblast* cells develop into new bone cells). The relative activity of these two types of cell are determined by local factors such as the loading applied to a particular bone and more general factors such as circulatory hormone concentrations. These factors ultimately determine tissue structure.

Mechanical strain, especially the rate of application of strain, appears to be a potent stimulus for bone growth. However, repetitive loading which stimulates osteoblast activity can also lead to damage in the form of micro-cracks[1] within bone (Martin and Burr 1982). Osteoclasts, in turn, will remove damaged material, thereby allowing osteoblasts to deposit matrix and minerals along the paths of applied stress (Carter 1984), forming new bone (Martin and Burr 1982). The high-volume training associated with middle and long-distance running may adversely influence these repair processes, in that bone is damaged at a faster rate than it is repaired (Bilanin, Blanchard and Russek-Cohen 1989). Changes in hormone concentrations associated with high training volumes exacerbate the problems caused by repetitive loading. In male runners, lowered testosterone and increased cortisol concentrations promote bone catabolism (Grimston *et al.* 1993). Similarly decreased oestradiol and increased prolactin concentrations in female runners contribute to reductions in bone mineral density (Chilibeck, Sale and Webber 1995).

The bone remodelling that takes place in response to an increase in training stress typically takes 8–12 weeks to stabilise. Thus, the runner would be most susceptible to bone tissue damage during this time, and would be advised to increase training volume in a gradual progression in order to allow time for bone to adapt to the new training stress.

EXERCISE-INDUCED METABOLIC (OXIDATIVE) STRESS

Exercise increases exposure to free radicals generated both within the body, and from external sources such as environmental pollution. Despite the potential for free radicals to produce tissue injury (McCord 1985, Halliwell and Chirico 1993, Diplock *et al.* 1998), they also perform a number of useful roles in body. For example, immune cells exploit the damaging effects of radicals to kill invading organisms such as bacteria, and to destroy tissue (Weiss 1989).

---

[1]Micro-cracks represent the initial injury to bone tissue, and their presence is normally imperceptible to the runner. However, these may develop over time into debilitating stress fractures.

Antioxidants protect tissues against the harmful effects of free radicals by decreasing their formation, converting these radicals to less reactive molecules and repairing oxidative tissue damage (Sen 1995). The principle antioxidants which a runner can obtain from their diet are the carotenoids (including β-carotene) and vitamins C and E. Zeaxanthin, β-cryptoxanthin and lycopene are carotenoids which occur naturally in vegetables such as carrots, tomatoes and spinach (Diplock *et al*. 1998). In some conditions these may be more effective at preventing free radical damage than β-carotene (Woodhall, Britton and Jackson 1997, Woodhall *et al*. 1997) and should therefore be considered as important contributors to antioxidant defences in humans.

The majority of the free radical protection within cells is thought to be provided by antioxidant enzymes, glutathione and carnosine (Bendich 1991, Sen 1995). Both glutathione (composed of the amino acids glutamine, cysteine and glycine) and carnosine (composed of the amino acids alanine and histidine) are produced in the body provided that the diet contains adequate levels of their precursor amino acids (Hunter and Grimble 1997). Outside the cell, vitamin C and uric acid take on a more important antioxidant role. The cellular distribution of non-enzymatic antioxidants is shown in Figure 7.2.

The rate of oxygen uptake from the lungs can increase 20-fold above resting values during race pace running. However, it is estimated that oxygen uptake by active muscle fibres may increase 200-fold (Keul, Doll and Koppler 1972). This increase in muscle metabolism appears to increase free radical formation (Davies *et al*. 1982, Jackson, Edwards and Symons 1985). Exercise-induced muscle ischaemia, where some muscle fibres have an inadequate blood supply, might also result in free radical formation (Witt *et al*. 1992, Packer 1997). However, available evidence in the scientific literature does not support this view (Mair *et al*. 1995, Jackson, McArdle and O'Farrel 1995) and the possibility that middle and long-distance runners experience ischaemic muscle injury is remote.

The physiological adaptations to training include an increase in the capacity of muscle to generate energy through aerobic oxidative metabolism. However, muscle antioxidant defences do not appear to increase at the same rate (Higuchi *et al*. 1985, Alessio and Goldfarb 1988, Gohil *et al*. 1987). Despite these apparent deficiencies in antioxidant protection, trained muscle is more resistant to oxidative damage than untrained muscle (Alessio and Goldfarb 1988). Thus, a rationale for dietary vitamin supplementation, based on the assumption that there is an increased susceptibility to oxidative injury in trained muscle, is not supported.

Although antioxidant supplementation might not be warranted at sea-level, there is evidence that vitamin E supplementation might be advantageous to the middle and long-distance runner whilst training or

mitochondrion

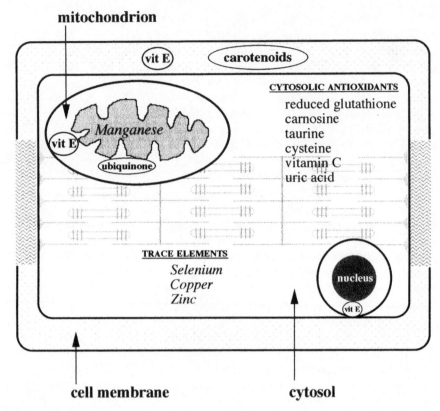

cell membrane   **cytosol**

Figure 7.2. Schematic diagram of the location of non-enzymatic antioxidants within a muscle fibre. The trace elements which enhance the activity of antioxidant enzymes are shown in italics. Selenium is a co-factor for glutathione peroxidase; copper and zinc are co-factors for cytosolic superoxide dismutase and manganese is a co-factor for mitochondrial superoxide dismutase.

competing at altitude (Ogawa 1970, Simon-Schnass and Pabst 1988). Chapter 9 describes the environmental challenge of the decrease in oxygen availability at altitude and the implications for exercise performance. Athletes taking a dietary vitamin E supplement equivalent to 300–400 mg day^{-1} at moderate altitude (1000 m above sea-level) were able to maintain $\dot{V}O_{2max}$ (Ogawa 1970) and sustain a higher percentage of $\dot{V}O_{2max}$ (Kobayashi 1974), in comparison with non-supplementing athletes. The mechanism by which supplementation improved aerobic performance is unclear, but may be due to improved capillary circulation (Simon-Schnass 1993) or increased free radical buffering. Either effect would help maintain optimal conditions for tissue functioning, even when oxygen availability was low.

LUNG INJURY

Lung ventilation can increase from around $10-12 \, l \, min^{-1}$ at rest, to over $140 \, l \, min^{-1}$ when running at middle-distance race pace. This increased ventilation will also increase the exposure of lung tissue to *ozone*, a toxic component of photochemical air pollution (Chapter 9). Aside from its direct toxic effects, ozone readily reacts with water (Mustafa 1990, Elstner and Osswald 1991) in the respiratory tract, producing highly reactive radicals (Glaze 1986). Thus, the potential for free radical damage to the respiratory tract would increase in proportion to increases in rate of oxygen uptake. Fortunately, the lining fluids of the respiratory tract contain a variety of antioxidants which help to minimise this damage (Cross *et al.* 1992). These antioxidants combine with inhaled ozone during its contact with the body's respiratory system, neutralising the radicals and thereby protecting sensitive regions of the lungs. Further protection might be offered by increasing the antioxidant defences of the actual cells lining the respiratory tract. Therefore, although lung tissue is exposed to increased free radical production during exercise, the antioxidant defences in non-smoking runners appear adequate.

RED BLOOD CELL DAMAGE

The primary role of red blood cells is to transport oxygen and carbon dioxide around the body. Thus, red blood cells undergo oxygenation in the lung and deoxygenation in the tissue, a process that is accelerated during exercise. This oxygenation–deoxygenation process results in free radical formation in red blood cells (Smith 1995, Gohil *et al.* 1987). As these events occur principally at the lung and skeletal muscle during exercise, both tissues could be exposed to the potentially harmful effects of red blood cell derived free radicals. A major site of damage from these free radicals is the red blood cell wall. This localised damage reduces the wall's flexibility and makes the cell more prone to breaking down during its passage around the vascular system, especially during the foot contact phase of running.

IMPLICATIONS FOR IMPROVING MIDDLE AND LONG-DISTANCE RUNNING PERFORMANCE

Training promotes a number of changes in the structure and function of several tissues which increases their resistance to mechanical and metabolic injury. Nevertheless, the tissues of well-conditioned middle and long-distance runners are still susceptible to exercise-induced damage. Strategies which minimise injury could optimise tissue functioning and thereby help maintain running performance.

Mechanical Damage

The mechanical damage associated with running primarily results from the high loadings imposed on the lower limbs during the foot contact phase. Thus, reductions in the loading rate (i.e. the strain rate) and loading stress (i.e. applied force per unit cross-sectional area of tissue) has the potential to reduce mechanically induced tissue injury. There are a number of strategies which might be employed to reduce the shock of impact during foot contact which range from the selection of appropriate footwear, to the choice of running surface and the type of training performed.

For more than a quarter of a century, it has been known that the use of rubber soled training shoes can reduce muscle damage during running (Buckle 1965), where midsole cushioning reduces the peak forces applied to tissues in the lower extremity. The usual penalty for improved musculoskeletal protection is increased running shoe weight, and a corresponding deterioration in running economy (Cavanagh and Kram 1985). In practical terms, training in a heavier shoe to minimise injury, and then competing in a lighter racing shoe to optimise competitive performance, might prove a sensible strategy. Selection of appropriate running shoes is perhaps an important first step to minimising mechanically induced tissue injuries. However, these shoes must be changed on a regular basis before their shock absorbent properties are lost. The forces applied to the lower limbs might be further reduced by running on compliant surfaces such as grass or sand, and avoiding less compliant surfaces such as concrete or tarmacadam.

Training *per se* offers some protection against the mechanical loadings which result in tissue damage, and the mechanisms of adaptation have been discussed previously. Training may also improve the fatigue resistance of muscles involved in attenuating the shock waves resulting from foot strike (e.g. *tibialis anterior* and *quadriceps*). Such adaptations, in turn, could reduce the peak impact forces and strain rates applied to the lower limbs, thus protecting other tissues from possible mechanical damage.

From a nutritional perspective, there is some evidence that vitamin C supplementation may assist in minimising mechanical damage by facilitating collagen formation (Peterkofsky 1991), thereby increasing connective tissue strength. However, excessive vitamin E supplementation has been shown to have some undesirable effects, being associated with increased susceptibility to oxidative damage in red blood cells (Brown,

Morrice and Duthie 1997). Thus, antioxidant supplementation may not always be beneficial to the middle and long-distance runner, as it has the potential to *promote* oxidative damage (especially when taken in high doses).

Hyperthermic and Ischaemic Gut Injury

Drinking strategies, which help maintain a runner's hydration status might decrease the incidence of exercise-induced gut complaints. This appears to be especially true in longer distance events such as the marathon, where only partial fluid replacement still reduces the rise in core temperature and contributes to the maintenance of running performance (refer to Chapter 9).

As discussed previously, gastrointestinal tract problems have been associated with the redistribution of blood flow during exercise, where blood flow to the abdomen is decreased and blood flow to skeletal muscle and skin is increased. One mechanism whereby fluid intake during exercise could reduce gut damage might be related to a reduction in the duration and severity of gut ischaemia. Thus, the damage associated with the restoration of normal blood flow following exercise would be reduced.

As well as supplementing with fluid to reduce ischaemic gut injury, a runner might also consider supplementing with the amino acid glutamine. The possible role of glutamine supplementation in enhancing immune function is discussed in Chapter 8; however increased glutamine availability to the gut is also associated with reduced susceptibility to ischaemic gut injury (Fijita and Sakurai 1995, Dugan and McBurney 1995). Possible mechanisms by which this might be achieved include increasing glutathione antioxidant protection of gut cells (where glutamine is an amino acid precursor to glutathione production), providing fuel for cell functioning and facilitating cell repair. The ideal glutamine supplementation programme is yet to be determined, but acute intakes of $2–8 \, g \, day^{-1}$ have been previously administered. However, porridge oats provide a good dietary source of glutamine.

The high incidence of traumatic injuries to soft tissues often leads a runner to use non-steroidal anti-inflammatory drug treatments (e.g. aspirin), which are known to produce gastric lesions. Therefore such treatments should be avoided during intense periods of training and competition, as they may exacerbate injury to cells lining the gut.

In addition to ischaemia, the gut might also be damaged during exercise by the jarring of its contents. One strategy to ease this problem would be to ensure that the weight of the gut contents during exercise is kept to a minimum. Brouns, Saris and Rehrer (1987) recommend that solid food should be avoided for the three hours preceding exercise. Moreover, runners who frequently experience exercise-related gastrointestinal problems might benefit from replacing their normal diet during the 24 hours pre-competition with a low fibre, nutritional liquid.

Metabolic Damage

The body's antioxidant defence against metabolic (oxidative) damage is not totally effective either at rest or during exercise. Race pace running increases the energy demand from aerobic metabolism and therefore increases the risk of free radical tissue damage. Orally administered antioxidant supplements have not been shown to improve running performance at sea level (Packer 1997). This failure of nutritional antioxidant supplements to influence performance suggests that the non-nutritional antioxidants already present in muscle (e.g. uric acid, glutathione, carnosine and muscle enzymes) are highly effective in minimising tissue injury and maintaining optimal tissue function in runners.

Many of the studies investigating the effects of antioxidant supplementation reported in the scientific literature have administered large amounts of individual antioxidants. It is becoming increasingly clear that the body's antioxidant defences are extremely complex, where single antioxidants work together in procuring their protective effect. Conversely, excessively high levels of individual antioxidants may produce detrimental effects (Brown, Morrice and Duthie 1997). Thus, increasing the intake of single antioxidants may not compensate for inadequacies in other areas of the antioxidant defences; moreover such an approach might prove detrimental by disturbing the antioxidant balance already present in tissue. It is therefore likely that the antioxidant requirements of middle and long-distance runners could be met from their daily diet without consuming supplements, providing it was high in fresh fruit and vegetables. Although nutritional strategies to reduce metabolic damage appear to have limited affect on running performance, other practical strategies have proved more successful.

Reducing free radical formation

Exercise increases free radical formation and therefore oxidative stress. Thus, decreasing activity levels prior to competition provides one mechanism by which oxidative stress might be reduced. Systematic reductions in training volume (i.e. training taper; refer to Chapter 5) can reduce muscle and oxidative injury during exercise (Child, Wilkinson and Fallowfield in press). This may result from allowing time for the antioxidant defences of cells to recover during the period of reduced training. A further consideration might be the environment in which a runner trains. Training in areas where air borne chemical pollutants are low would further reduce pre-competition oxidative stress, and hence help to ensure that antioxidant defences are optimal prior to competition.

Interception of free radicals with antioxidants

Increasing tissue antioxidant levels, so that free radicals formed during exercise are readily intercepted, provides another mechanism by which oxidative stress might be minimised. Fortunately for the middle and long-distance runner, aerobic training *per se* produces many physiological adaptations which enhance cellular antioxidant defences. As discussed previously, identification of dietary antioxidant supplements which complement the body's natural defences have proved elusive. Nevertheless, the best therapeutic results appear to be achieved when a supplementation strategy considers all the components in the antioxidant chain (Sen 1995). At a relatively simplistic level, one approach might be to administer a multivitamin supplement. An *ideal* supplement would combine vitamins C and E with enzyme co-factors, such as selenium and zinc, along with a spectrum of carotenoids. It should be noted that despite the fact that iron supplements are commonly taken by middle and long-distance runners to address compromised iron status (Chapter 8), they should not be taken concurrent with supplements containing vitamin C. This is because iron combines with vitamin C, increasing free radical production in the gut. One strategy might be to take the supplement containing vitamin C early in the day, and then to take the iron supplement with the evening meal.

Increasing cell wall (membrane) resistance to oxidation

The membranes of cells, including muscle cells (fibres) and cell organelles (the functional components of cells), contain chemicals referred to as fatty acids. Fatty acids are discussed in greater detail in Chapter 8; within the context of the present discussion they can be differentiated on the basis of their chemical structure (i.e. polyunsaturated, monounsaturated and saturated). The fatty acids contained within a runner's diet will partly influence their composition within cell membranes (Robblee and Clandinin 1984). Thus, cellular membranes in a runner consuming a diet rich in polyunsaturated fatty acids will largely be made up of polyunsaturated fatty acids. Conversely, the cellular membranes in runners consuming a diet rich in either monounsaturated or saturated fatty acids will generally comprise either monounsaturated or saturated fatty acids respectively.

Saturated fats are totally resistant to oxidative damage; nevertheless a diet high in saturated fats cannot be advocated due to the adverse implications for general health. Monounsaturated fats are more resistant to oxidative damage than polyunsaturated fats, and increasing their intake in the daily diet (e.g. foods rich in monounsaturated fats include olive oil, avocados, cashew nuts, hazelnuts and almonds) might enhance the intrinsic resistance of cell membranes to oxidative damage. Such a strategy might be appropriate for a runner in the months prior to and during intensive periods of training and competition.

SUMMARY

Poor management of training, such as sudden changes in training mileage, training intensity or failing to allow sufficient time for recovery, are the primary causes of injury amongst runners (James, Bates and Osternig 1978, Janssen and ten Hoor 1989). Recovery is essential, both in terms of the rest intervals between training sessions and the recovery following exercise-related tissue injuries. Finding a suitable training programme that facilitates maximum training gains, whilst preventing an accumulation in tissue damage, is extremely difficult. Perhaps in the competitive world of middle and long-distance running, the successful runners might consider focusing upon minimising tissue damage as one approach to optimising race performance.

KEY POINTS

- Paradoxically, training for middle and long-distance running initially causes tissue damage before resulting in performance-enhancing adaptations.
- For optimal training gains to be made, a runner must find their individual balance between applying the training stimulus and allowing sufficient recovery time for repair and adaptation to occur.
- The most damaging mechanisms through which tissue becomes damaged are ischaemia, hyperthermia, metabolic stress and mechanical loading.
- The principal sites of damage during middle and long-distance running are musculoskeletal soft tissue, bone, red blood cells and gut.
- Mechanically induced soft tissue injuries can result in inflammation. When this occurs, the training load must be reduced to avoid potentially more chronic re-injury.
- A runner is most susceptible to bone tissue damage during the initial

8–12 weeks following an increase in training stress. Therefore training volume should be gradually increased in order to avoid debilitating bone damage.

- Muscle free radical production is increased in trained runners. However, their antioxidant defences appear more than adequate to cope, and the use of nutritional antioxidant supplements may not be warranted.
- The body's antioxidant defences are extremely complex, and single antioxidant supplements may disturb the antioxidant balance already present in tissue. Therefore, combination supplements combining vitamins C and E with selenium, zinc and a spectrum of carotenoids might prove more beneficial.
- Injury to gut tissue, which may contribute to exercise-related gastrointestinal problems, could be minimised by adopting an appropriate fluid intake strategy before, during and after exercise; minimising the weight of the gut contents during exercise; and, possibly by supplementing with glutamine.
- Middle and long-distance runners who wish to avoid long injury layoffs from competition should adopt a progressive training programme which considers minimising tissue damage as well as maximising training gain.

Chapter 8

Nutrition for Performance

Joanne L. Fallowfield

INTRODUCTION

Over the last 50 years, the importance of appropriate nutrition in maximising the body's athletic potential has been increasingly recognised. The sports science literature has clearly demonstrated a link between what the runner eats and how they perform (Bergstrom, Hermansen and Saltin 1967, Karlsson and Saltin 1971). Eating a sound sports diet is not going to make you run faster, rather it will enable race pace to be maintained for longer and therefore improve average sustainable running speed. The benefits of optimum sports nutrition are not experienced through a snatched healthy option just prior to competition, nor are they the result of popping the latest nutrient pill, but rather they are reflected in habitual eating habits. The basic message is very simple: a balanced diet for life provides the foundation for an optimum sports diet. The needs of middle and long-distance runners are qualitatively similar to those of the average man or woman, although quantitatively there may be a few differences.

A healthy, well-balanced diet must contain the right amounts of a number of essential nutrients. In terms of providing the body with fuel, carbohydrates and fats are the most important with protein providing no more than 6–10% of the total energy for exercise. Vitamins and minerals are only required in relatively small amounts, but must be provided in the diet on a daily basis. Fibre, also referred to as non-starch polysaccharide (NSP), is a necessary component of the diet that is largely composed of the major constituents of plant cell walls (e.g. cellulose, pectins, glucans, arabinogalactons, gums, mucilages and chitin). These constituents can be absorbed into the body from the large intestine where they are fermented by anaerobic flora.

Fibre performs a number of essential roles including: adding bulk to food, so reducing the temptation to over-eat; helping to smooth the passage of food along the gastrointestinal tract; facilitating the transport and absorption of other essential nutrients; aiding the retention of water in faeces; and improving the excretion of toxins from the large intestine. A diet deficient in fibre is associated with digestive problems such as constipation, gall stones and bowel disorders. Cereals, grains (e.g. bread, breakfast cereals, rice and pasta), fruit, vegetables and potatoes (especially baked in their skins) are all good sources of fibre. Finally, the importance of water in the diet cannot be over-stated. Water performs a central structural role (over 60% of the body's mass is fluid) but is also essential in the body's main transport system and in the regulation of body temperature. These issues will be further addressed in Chapter 9.

THE RUNNER'S ENERGY REQUIREMENTS

The runner's diet must provide between approximately 1800 and 4000 kcal[1] of energy every day, depending upon such factors as training status, training volume, male or female, body size, an individual's rate of metabolism and possibly age. Ideally, at least 60% of this energy should be in the form of carbohydrates (e.g. potatoes, rice, pasta, sugars and fruit), no more than 25% in the form of fats (e.g. oils, butter, cheese) and the remaining 15% as protein (e.g. fish and lean meat).

The most important dietary energy provider for the runner, carbohydrate, is present in the diet as chains of sugar units, where each unit is made up of carbon, hydrogen and oxygen molecules. The process of digestion breaks down these chains into shorter lengths of sugar units. Dietary carbohydrates can be classified as either mono-, di- or polysaccharides, depending upon their chain length. Examples of monosaccharides (i.e. single units) are fructose or fruit sugar, glucose and galactose. Disaccharides are formed by the linking of two monosaccharides; for example, sucrose is a combination of glucose and fructose. The linking of many monosaccharides by chemical bonds gives rise to polysaccharides such as the starch which is found in plant food.

---

[1]The *calorie* is the most commonly used unit of energy but is relatively small, therefore the *kilocalorie* is more frequently used (1 kcal = 1000 calories). Energy values cited in the text will normally be presented in kcal. However, the *joule* is a more contemporary unit for measuring energy that often appears on modern food packaging labels; 1 joule is the energy expended when 1 kilogramme is moved 1 meter by a force of 1 Newton. An approximate conversion of kilocalories to kilojoules is given by: 1 kcal = 4.2 kJ.

Carbohydrate foods are often discussed in terms of whether they contain predominantly simple carbohydrates (sugars such as fruit juices, milk, yoghurt, honey and jam) or complex carbohydrates (starches in potatoes, rice, bread, pasta, porridge oats and beans). Such a classification may be somewhat confusing as most foods contain a mixture of both simple and complex carbohydrates (e.g. breakfast cereals). The glycaemic index (GI) reflects the time course of blood glucose availability following ingestion (Jenkins *et al*. 1981). Factors which influence the GI of a food include: biochemical structure; rate of absorption in the intestine; the size of the food particles; the degree of thermal processing; the content and timing of the previous meal; and the co-ingestion of fat, protein or fibre (Guezennec 1995). Foods with a high GI are rapidly digested and absorbed by the body, and therefore are more readily available to the runner for fuelling exercise. Table 8.1 lists some examples of high, moderate and low glycaemic foods. Thus, a more contemporary view would be to consider: the GI of the food; the nutritional package of that food and how it contributes to the overall diet; the availability of that food; and its taste. All these factors will influence the development of a high carbohydrate diet, and not simply whether a food contains sugar or starch.

In addition to providing energy for exercise and acting as a medium for the absorption of various micronutrients from the small intestine (e.g. fat-soluble vitamins), fat performs a number of essential structural, functional and regulatory roles. Nevertheless, it is a nutrient that many middle and long-distance runners will religiously avoid. The majority of dietary fats are composed of triglycerides, which following digestion are absorbed as chains of carbon, hydrogen and oxygen (i.e. fatty acids) and as an alcohol (i.e. glycerol).

Fatty acids are either saturated or unsaturated[2], depending upon their chemical structure. Saturated fats are mainly found in animal foods such as meats and dairy products. These foods are also sources of cholesterol, which plays a number of structural roles in the body, in addition to forming the basis of a number of hormones, vitamin D and bile. It is not necessary for the diet to provide cholesterol since the body is able to manufacture adequate amounts of cholesterol to fulfil its needs. Foods containing vegetable oils (e.g. olive oil, sunflower oil, rape seed oil and corn oil) are good sources of unsaturated fats, which

---

[2]Saturated fats, which are usually solid at room temperature, contain only a single multiple bond between the constituent molecules and therefore have limited scope for undergoing further chemical reactions. In contrast, unsaturated fats contain one or more double or triple bonds and are therefore able to incorporate additional hydrogen atoms. Unsaturated fats are usually liquid (oil) at room temperature.

Table 8.1. Examples of carbohydrate (CHO) containing foods with high, moderate and low glycaemic indexes (foods listed as eaten)

Food group	Food item	Serving size providing 50 g of CHO (g or ml)	Fat per serving (g)
High glycaemic index			
Cereals	White bread	201 g	2
	Wholemeal bread	120 g	3
Breakfast cereals	Corn flakes	59 g	1
	Muesli	76 g	6
Biscuit	Wholewheat biscuit	76 g	16
Vegetables	Sweet corn	219 g	5
	Broad beans	704 g	4
	Potatoes (boiled)	254 g	trace
Fruit	Raisins	78 g	trace
	Banana	260 g	1
Sugars	Glucose	50 g	0
	Maltose	50 g	0
	Honey	67 g	3
	Sucrose	50 g	0
Beverages	6% Sucrose solution	833 ml	0
	7.5% Maltodextrin and sugar	666 ml	0
	10% Carbonated soft drink	500 ml	0
	20% Maltodextrin	250 ml	0
Moderate glycaemic index			
Cereals	Spaghetti/macaroni	198 g	1
	Noodles (oriental)	370 g	14
Breakfast cereals	Wheat bran	232 g	13
	Oatmeal	69 g	1
Biscuits	Oatmeal biscuits	79 g	15
	Sponge cake	93 g	6
Fruit	Grapes (black)	323 g	trace
	Grapes (green)	310 g	trace
	Orange	420–600 g	trace
Low glycaemic index			
Fruits	Apples	400 g	trace
	Cherries	420 g	trace
	Dates (dried)	78 g	trace
	Peaches	450–550 g	trace
	Plums	400–550 g	trace
Sugars	Fructose	50 g	0
Dairy products	Ice cream	202 g	13
	Milk (whole)	1100 ml	40
	Milk (skimmed)	1000 ml	1
	Yoghurt (plain, low fat)	800 g	8
	Yoghurt (fruit, low fat)	280 g	3
Soup	Tomato soup	734 ml	6

Adapted from Coyle (1991).

contain varying amounts of poly- and monounsaturated fatty acids. Runners should aim to make a moderate fat intake their goal; Table 8.2 provides a general guide for estimating an appropriate daily fat intake. A fat intake of less than 30 g per day (g day^{-1}) may compromise the provision of fat-soluble vitamins and essential fatty acids necessary to maintain good health.

Protein only covers a relatively small fraction of the body's energy needs under normal circumstances. The main function of dietary protein is concerned with growth and repair, especially following strenuous exercise. Under extreme circumstances, such as during the latter stages of ultra-distance running, a runner will increasingly call upon protein in muscle to fuel exercise performance. Protein is made up of amino acid building blocks, and aside from the protein structurally incorporated into the body, there is no discrete amino acid store. The daily protein requirement of an endurance runner is equivalent to 1.2–1.4 g kg^{-1} body weight per day (Lemon 1991), which equates to approximately 85 g of protein in total per day. Refer to Table 8.3 for some examples of foods which provide 25 g of protein per serving as detailed. An excessively high protein intake would not be advantageous to the runner; the breakdown of proteins during energy metabolism results in the release of nitrogen in the form of ammonia, which in high concentrations can become toxic. Under normal circumstances, the ammonia resulting from protein breakdown is converted to urea in the liver and excreted by the kidneys. Therefore, a diet exceptionally high in protein may be associated with kidney problems, though this is yet to be scientifically proven.

Refer to the Appendix for some meal plan ideas. Examples are given of high-carbohydrate breakfasts, snacks, light meals and main meals. These should not be used as definitive menus, but rather they should provide

Table 8.2. Conversion of the percentage of total energy intake into grammes of fat

Total dietary energy intake (kcal)	20–30% energy intake as fat range (g)
1800	40–60
2000	44–66
2500	55–83
3000	66–100
3500	77–116
4000	88–113
4500	100–150
5000	111–166

Table 8.3. Food servings providing 25 g protein

Food	Portion size (g)	Household serving
Meat, fish, eggs		
Chicken	100	Breast
Lean meat (sliced)	100	4 medium slices
Minced meat	100	2 large tablespoons
Steak	125	1 medium
Tinned fish	100	0.5 can
Fresh fish	100–200	1 steak
Prawns	150	1 mug
Eggs (boiled)	100	2 eggs
Dairy produce		
Milk	500	1 pint; 0.5 litre
Cheese	100	2 small matchboxes
Fruit yoghurt	450	3 cartons
Bread and buns		
Bread (toast)	300	6 thick slices
Bread rolls/buns/English muffins	250	5 items
Pizza (deep pan)	250	2 slices
Pasta, rice, potatoes, noodles		
Pasta (uncooked)	200	10 tablespoons
Rice (uncooked)	300	12 tablespoons
Potatoes (boiled)	1600	16 medium potatoes
Breakfast cereals (plus half a pint of milk)		
Sweetened	200	12 tablespoons
Unsweetened	100	8 tablespoons
Muesli (sweetened)	100	3 tablespoons
Fruit, vegetables, beans		
Bananas/apples/oranges/vegetables		Negligible
Beans	500	6 tablespoons
Other		
Nuts	100	1 medium packet
Seeds	150	4–6 tablespoons
Lentils	100	4 tablespoons

guidance for runners to structure their own dietary day to meet their lifestyle needs.

THE VEGETARIAN RUNNER

There is no nutritional reason why a vegetarian runner should be at a disadvantage in comparison with their meat-eating counterparts, providing that the meat and fish (and dairy products if following a vegan diet) that have been omitted are replaced with an appropriate alternative (e.g.

beans, lentils, peas, nuts, tofu, quorn, etc.). Thus, a vegetarian runner will need to think a little more carefully when organising their nutritional day. The main area of attention should be focused upon the *quality* of protein, which refers to its amino acid content. Most of the amino acids which are required can be manufactured within the body from other amino acids (i.e. non-essential amino acids). However, there are eight essential amino acids which must be provided by the daily diet.

Animal sources of protein (e.g. meat, fish, eggs, milk, yoghurt and cheese) are relatively rich in essential amino acids. In contrast, vegetable sources of protein may not provide all the essential amino acids in a single serving. This will necessitate the combining of vegetable foods over the course of the day to ensure that the body receives all the essential amino acids. Some sources of vegetable protein (e.g. soya beans and related products) contain a more complete range of these essential amino acids and it would therefore be appropriate to include these foods on the menu at some point during the day (e.g. replacing meat with a soya bean alternative).

In addition to ensuring a good balance of the essential amino acids in their diet, vegetarian runners must also be careful in selecting foods providing adequate sources of vitamin A, riboflavin, vitamin B_{12}, vitamin D, calcium, iron and zinc, and sufficient calories to meet their daily energy demands. It is always preferable for the runner to eat foods containing these important nutrients rather than turning to supplementary pills and powders. Dairy products are good sources of calcium, vitamin B_{12} and riboflavin. The situation is more complex for vegan runners; dark leafy vegetables, yeast, beans, lentils, nuts, soya products, quorn and foods fortified with vitamins may help to avoid any potential deficiencies. If a vegetarian runner, especially a recent convert, is experiencing a sustained deterioration in performance that cannot be traced to a problem in training, it might be wise to consult a qualified sports dietician or sports nutritionist to assess the adequacy (or otherwise) of their diet and dietary practices.

FOOD TO FUEL

As discussed in Chapter 3, the contraction of a muscle can only be fuelled directly by the chemical adenosine triphosphate (ATP). The runner, therefore, has to convert food eaten in their diet to ATP in order to power muscle contractions. Hence, ATP is often referred to as the *universal currency of free energy*, in that it is manufactured from carbohydrates, fats and proteins. The first stage in the process of liberating the chemical energy stored in food is digestion, where larger compounds are broken down into much smaller molecules which can readily be absorbed from the intestine. For example, the starch in potatoes and rice is broken down into smaller sugar units of monosaccharides or disaccharides, the fat in cheese or milk is broken down into fatty acids and glycerol, and the protein in meat and fish is broken down into smaller peptide chains or individual amino acids. Following absorption, glucose units, fatty acids and some amino acids are either used directly by muscle in biochemical processes which manufacture ATP, or are transported to discrete locations around the body for storage in the case of carbohydrates and fats, or further metabolism in the case of proteins.

The major carbohydrate stores are located in muscle and liver, where monosaccharides are joined together to form a long, branching, chain-like structure called glycogen. Glycogen is a relatively inefficient storage medium as it is laid down in a one-to-three parts ratio with water (Sherman *et al*. 1982). A high water content reduces the energy density of the carbohydrate stores, which amount to approximately 2000 kcal (i.e. approximately 500 g of carbohydrate) of energy in the average runner. This absolute figure will depend upon such factors as a runner's training status and their habitual diet, specifically the carbohydrate content of their diet (Sherman and Costill 1984). These finite carbohydrate stores may prove limiting during prolonged running, being adequate to fuel moderate-intensity exercise (i.e. equivalent to 70–75% $\dot{V}O_{2max}$) for around 90 minutes (Costill 1988).

In contrast, fat is an extremely efficient energy storage medium. The main reserves are located under the skin, packed around vital organs, or in discrete gender-specific fat depots. As a consequence of this body-wide distribution, even the leanest distance runners will have relatively inexhaustible fat reserves. The total energy stored as fat may exceed 100 000 kcal of energy in the average runner, which is theoretically enough to complete nearly forty sub-2:40:00 marathon races back to back! Such a feat may be beyond even the very best ultra-distance runners, so the question to be addressed concerns what limits endurance performance from an energy provision perspective.

FUELLING THE RUNNER

Exercising muscles are indirectly powered by a mixture of carbohydrates and fats. The rates at which these fuels can be converted to ATP depends upon the respective biochemical processes involved. The release of ATP from carbohydrates is a relatively fast process (high ATP power) but as mentioned previously the body's stores of carbohydrate are limited (low ATP capacity). In contrast, fats take longer to yield ATP (low ATP power), but their stores are much greater (high ATP capacity). The intensity of exercise, and the duration of exercise, will determine which fuel is predominantly used by the runner, though other issues such as training status and local environmental conditions will also play a part.

During rest and light exercise, fat can provide energy at a rate to cover most of the body's demands. As exercise intensity increases, energy in the form of ATP must be made available to working muscles at a higher rate. Carbohydrate can provide ATP more rapidly than fat and, as a consequence, is the preferred fuel for intense periods of hard running. During very intense bursts of activity (e.g. at the start of a race or during a sprint finish), muscles may draw upon stores of the high-energy phosphate, phosphocreatine. However, phosphocreatine stores are very small, such that very high intensity running, or sprinting, may only be sustained for several seconds.

The average club runner will expend between 0.21 and 0.30 kcal $min^{-1} kg^{-1}$ body weight whilst exercising. Thus, during a 1500 m race this would equate to a little over 100 kcal of energy, over 300 kcal of energy during a 5000 m race, over 600 kcal during a 10 000 m race and over 3000 kcal of energy during a marathon. Obviously, these absolute values will depend upon the body weight of the runner, training status, the conditions under foot (e.g. track versus road), prevailing environmental conditions and the runner's relative exercise intensity. From the previous discussion, this total energy requirement will be met in the main from both carbohydrate and fat reserves. However, it is the replenishment of the body's carbohydrate stores which is of paramount importance following training or competition.

HIGH-CARBOHYDRATE VERSUS HIGH-FAT DIETS

The basic diet of a middle and long-distance runner needs to provide all the essential nutrients for optimum health, though the total energy intake will normally have to be increased to accommodate high training volumes. The factors influencing the absolute energy requirements have been discussed earlier in this chapter; however in recent years there has been some anecdotal and scientific evidence to suggest that active individuals might benefit from increasing their total energy intake through the consumption of additional fat rather than additional carbohydrates (Lambert *et al.* 1994, Lapachet, Miller and Arnall 1996, Muoio *et al.* 1994, Van Zyl *et al.* 1996). Specifically, it has been suggested that ultra-endurance athletes should ingest a high-fat diet (i.e. 60–70% of kcal) for two to four weeks prior to competition, and then change to a high-carbohydrate diet approximately two days before the event.

The rationale for such a strategy is two-fold: first, an athlete should increase their readily available intra-muscular fat reserves prior to competition (i.e. the fat stores located in close proximity to the muscle fibres); and second, through associated metabolic muscle adaptations to a high-fat diet (i.e. increased enzyme activity), fat oxidation during exercise might be increased whilst oxidation of the finite carbohydrate reserves is reduced (Phinney *et al.* 1983). Such a simplistic *supply and demand* approach to energy metabolism, whilst essentially sound, assumes that if the muscle is provided with greater quantities of an alternate fuel it will actually be able to utilise this fuel in preference to carbohydrate. However, in practice, fat oxidation does not normally support sustained exercise at intensities of greater than approximately 50% VO_{2max}.

The relative contribution of fat metabolism to fuelling exercise might be further improved by the co-ingestion of micro-nutrients such as caffeine. Caffeine increases the mobilisation and availability of free fatty acids, and hence their subsequent oxidation in generating energy (Costill *et al.* 1977). In addition, aerobic training is also regarded as having a favourable lipolytic[3] effect, being associated with increases in the mobilisation and metabolism of fats (Coggan and Williams 1995). Nevertheless, increasing dietary fat in excess of approximately 30% of total energy intake tends to be associated with a counter-productive reduction in dietary carbohydrate intake, and a commensurate inability to maintain muscle glycogen reserves prior to competition (Sherman and Leenders 1995). A further consideration to add to this high-fat versus high-carbohydrate diet debate would be the long-term health implications of extreme dietary modifications, where high-fat diets have been associated with an increased risk of coronary heart disease, stroke and certain cancers. Thus, despite the tremendous speculation in the popular sports press, there is presently no sound scientific evidence to support the use of high-fat diets to improve middle and long-distance running performance (Sherman and Leenders 1995). However there may be a case for their cautious use in preparing for ultra-endurance events.

FUEL FOR TRAINING

No amount of quality training will ensure a winning performance on race day if the runner fails to refuel after each exercise bout. An engine will not run if the fuel tank is empty and the same is true of the human

---

[3]Lipolysis refers to the breakdown of fats to fatty acids and glycerol; therefore aerobic training is one strategy for improving this process in the runner.

engine. Replenishing the body's energy reserves may take place during a training session with an appropriately formulated sports drink in the feeding bottle, although the greater part will take place after exercise. The post-training diet needs to be planned with the same meticulous attention to detail as is paid to the actual training session itself. It is important that time is made to re-fuel prior to further bouts of exercise. In the short term, a runner in energy deficit will experience a reduced training gain, whilst also being susceptible to injury or illness. Of greater concern is the potential link between a runner being in a sustained glycogen-depleted state and the incidence of prolonged fatigue syndrome, over-reaching or overtraining syndrome (Lehmann, Foster and Keul 1993) (Chapter 5).

A typical sports diet will contain from 300 to 400 g of carbohydrate (equivalent to between 4.5 and 5.0 g kg^{-1} body weight). However, this has been shown to be inadequate for replenishing the glycogen stores of a runner in regular training on a daily basis (Costill *et al.* 1971a). Thus, an increased dietary carbohydrate intake of from 500 to 600 g (8.0 to 9.0 g kg^{-1} body weight) of carbohydrate is recommended (Costill *et al.* 1981, Fallowfield and Williams 1993). It should be noted that during intensive periods of high-volume training, an intake of greater than 700 g of carbohydrate (9.0 to 10.0 g kg^{-1} body weight) may be necessary. Table 8.4 provides some suggestions of high-carbohydrate foods which could be incorporated into a training diet. Care should be taken that the accompanying dishes ensure that the eating plan is balanced with respect to all of the essential nutrients.

PREPARING FOR COMPETITION

In preparing for competition, the golden rule is never to try anything new on race day. Training should provide an opportunity to rehearse race day strategies in addition to ensuring that the body is at its physical and psychological peak.

During the season, depending upon the specialist distance of the runner, it is likely that they will race most weekends and possibly midweek as well. With other commitments such as family and work, this will relegate training to the twilight hours with eating fitting in when (and if) possible. Special consideration must be given to the planning of a dietary schedule, together with a training and competition schedule. Refuelling the body is too important to be left as an afterthought. The details of a runner's preparation for competition should be tailored to their personal situation, but will generally depend upon such factors as: the duration of recovery required by the body between races; the position of the race with respect to a runner's focus

Table 8.4. Food servings providing 50 g carbohydrate

Food	Portion size (g)	Household serving
Bread and buns		
Bread/toast	100	2 thick slices
Baguette	100	1 medium piece
Pitta bread/bagels	100	1 large
Bread rolls/buns/scones	100	2 pieces
Pasta/rice/potatoes/noodles		
Pasta (uncooked)	75 (dry weight)	3–4 tablespoons
Rice (uncooked)	75 (dry weight)	3 tablespoons
Noodles (uncooked)	75 (dry weight)	1 sheet
Potatoes (boiled)	300	2–3 pieces
Sweet potatoes	250	3 pieces
Jacket potatoes	200	1 large
Couscous (dry weight)	150 (dry weight)	6 tablespoons
Breakfast cereals (plus half a pint of milk)		
Sweetened cereals	50	3–4 tablespoons*
Muesli (sweetened)	75	2 tablespoons*
Wholegrain cereals	75	6–8 tablespoons*
Porridge	400	1 large bowl
Fruit/vegetables/beans		
Bananas	300	2 large
Apples	500	3 pieces
Oranges	800	5 pieces
Raisins	50	1 handful
Beans	300	3 tablespoons*
Tinned fruit	300	3 tablespoons*
Fruit juice	500	0.5 litre (1.0 pint)
Dairy produce		
Milk (skimmed)	1000	1.0 litre (2.0 pints)

*These are generous tablespoons piled with the food.
Nutrient data from Paul and Southgate (1978).

for the season; and the importance with which the race is personally rated.

In longer duration races, such as half and full marathons, where the event lasts in excess of 60 minutes and the body's stores of carbohydrate may become limiting, performance may benefit from some form of dietary *carbohydrate loading* regime. Traditionalists will profess the virtues of the classic seven-day carbohydrate loading strategy initially advocated by Scandinavian exercise scientists in the 1960s (Åstrand 1967). This involves a strenuous training session approximately one week prior to race day, where the aim is to lower muscle glycogen stores. This is followed by a three-day depletion phase, where the runner consumes a diet low in carbohydrates with additional energy as required from fat and protein. Finally, over the four days leading up to the race, the runner systematically reduces their training volume (i.e. training taper; refer to Chapter 5) whilst consuming a high-carbohydrate diet.

There is no doubt that this strategy does increase the muscles' carbohydrate stores prior to competition (Karlsson and Saltin 1971), but this may be at a price (Costill and Miller 1980). First, there is always an element of risk associated with a hard, exhaustive training session performed so close to a major event, where the danger may be a careless injury or excessive fatigue from which recovery takes longer than planned. Second, the further potential for injury as a consequence of continuing to train in a fatigued, glycogen-depleted state is high. Finally, the depletion phase may also be associated with irritability, headaches, lethargy and a poor psychological state of mind with respect to the imminent race, as a consequence of the body's depressed carbohydrate stores.

During the 1980s a more runner-friendly approach to carbohydrate supercompensation was shown to be equally as effective in optimising the body's glycogen stores (Sherman *et al.* 1981). This approach did not require the injury potentiating, hard training session close to competition, neither did it require a runner to follow a restricted diet whilst continuing to train at a normal level. The contemporary approach combines training taper with a high carbohydrate diet (9.0 to 10.0 g CHO kg^{-1} body weight). When followed over the seven days prior to competition (i.e. seven to four days prior to race day, 50% of total energy intake in the form of carbohydrates, increasing carbohydrate content to 70% of total energy intake over the last three days), this strategy similarly ensured that the carbohydrate stores of muscle were elevated, whilst avoiding the problems associated with the classic approach.

Despite the undoubted benefits of supercompensating the body's limited fuel reserves through *carbo-loading*, there are a few negative consequences of which a runner needs to be aware in order to make an informed decision. As discussed previously, the body lays down glycogen in association with water. Consequently there is a possibility that the body will feel heavier at the start of a race, whilst the muscles may feel a little stiff. In terms of performance, a carbohydrate-loaded runner may therefore be slower in terms of absolute running speed over the early stages of a race. However, this stiffness will start to wear off as the body mobilises its glycogen stores, and a runner may reap the rewards in the latter stages of the race as they are able to maintain race pace when fellow competitors start to fade. This latter point highlights the fact that carbohydrate loading will only be a useful aid to competition in events where the availability of endogenous[4] carbohydrate stores become limiting (e.g. half-marathon in slower runners, marathon and ultra-endurance races). If there is not a deficiency, providing more carbohydrate will not improve race performance.

For most long-distance runners, for whom a carbohydrate loading strategy might be appropriate, it is difficult to accommodate the luxury of such a pre-race build-up during a busy season. Nevertheless, there are a few general guidelines to preparation which may hold some benefits for performance. A runner should always ensure that they take appropriate action to ensure that their muscle and liver glycogen stores are well stocked during the three days leading up to a race. Select meals high in carbohydrates, providing the body with its readily available energy substrate in addition to the requisite vitamins and minerals to balance the diet. A high-carbohydrate diet may be supplemented with—not replaced by—an appropriately formulated sports drink; whilst providing additional carbohydrate, this approach would help reduce the *volume* of the diet, especially for runners who are not big eaters. In addition, taper training to avoid drawing heavily upon these fuel reserves and consciously increase fluid intake to effectively over-hydrate the body.

REFUELLING DURING EXERCISE

In middle-distance running there do not appear to be any significant performance benefits to be obtained by taking on additional fuel and fluid during a race. As with any nutritional supplement, carbohydrate will only aid performance if there is a deficiency; that is, if the demands of skeletal muscle are in excess of the body's capacity to supply. Assuming a runner has followed the simple guidelines to optimise muscle glycogen prior to competition, carbohydrate availability will not limit middle-distance race performance. However, this situation becomes very different during longer races, notably the half-marathon and marathon, for reasons discussed previously in this chapter. It has been shown that ingesting carbohydrate-containing beverages during such events enables a runner to maintain their optimal pace for longer in the race (Tsintzas *et al.* 1993, Williams *et al.* 1990).

The need, and desire, to take on additional fuel and fluids during a race will depend upon the specific course profile, local environmental conditions and the tactical nature of the race. The opportunity to refuel is

---

[4]Endogenous refers to substances occurring within the body, in contrast to supplementary carbohydrate which is exogenous or from outside the body.

generally dictated by the race regulations in terms of the location of feeding stations and the type of drink provided. Often in these circumstances the drink provided for the *masses* is plain water or dilute fruit cordials. If you are not in the fortunate position of being able to locate your personal feeding bottle at drinks' stations, it is worth remembering that even plain water can help reduce the rate of glycogen depletion in exercising muscle (Hargreaves *et al.* 1996) and improve endurance running capacity (Fallowfield *et al.* 1996). However, in training, problems of fluid availability and appropriateness of the fluid for a runner's particular needs should not arise, and it would be wise to ensure that feeding takes place throughout a session where possible.

The most readily absorbed *feeds* are dilute (2–8%[5]) carbohydrate solutions. There are numerous very good sports drinks now available on the market; however those providing carbohydrate in a form that keeps the osmolality (i.e. the ratio of solutes to fluid) of the beverage low and containing a small quantity of electrolytes (principally sodium) appear to work best. Both the carbohydrate and the electrolytes aid the processes by which a drink moves through the stomach and into the intestine (Maughan 1991). There is also a mechanical effect of the drink on these processes that is dictated by the feeding pattern. For example, drinking little and often (between 100 and 150 ml of fluid every 10 min, or the equivalent of a 500 ml feeding bottle every hour) will promote the movement of a drink through the stomach, and facilitate its subsequent availability for absorption in the intestine (Rehrer *et al.* 1990). It is only when a solution is in the small intestine that it can be absorbed by the body and is then available to fuel running performance. This volume of fluid may at first appear relatively high and may also initially be associated with a degree of gastrointestinal discomfort. However, a runner's tolerance to drinking during exercise can normally be trained, such that any feelings of discomfort would ease over time.

Once in the body, the exogenous carbohydrate supplements the body's finite reserves, whereas the role of the electrolytes principally enhances absorption of the fluid from the intestine and subsequent retention in the body. Specifically, electrolytes help in maintaining a *hydratory balance*; the addition of sodium to a sports drink decreases urine production in comparison to when a runner drinks plain water. It might also be argued that electrolytes are lost during exercise as salt in sweat, and hence one might speculate that they will need to be replaced. However, under

---

[5]The percentage carbohydrate content of a beverage represents the number of grammes per 100 ml of fluid (i.e. concentration of the fluid). For example, a dilute 2% solution would contain 2 g of carbohydrate per 100 ml of fluid.

normal temperate race conditions this loss is not thought to be detrimental to performance (Maughan 1991). Only in very extreme environmental conditions are the use of salt tablets or other saline replacement media advocated, and usually only under the guidance of a medical physician. The issue of fluid and electrolyte balance will be discussed in greater detail in Chapter 9.

RECOVERING FROM TRAINING AND COMPETITION

At the end of a training session or following competition, the sooner the refuelling process can be initiated the better. Delaying carbohydrate ingestion over this immediate post-exercise period has been demonstrated to delay recovery significantly (Ivy *et al.* 1988a) and hence extend the time interval when a runner is unable to perform optimally. The intensity and duration of the previous exercise bout will also influence the recovery process, such that greater attention to refuelling needs to be taken when the runner has been involved in a long, intense training session or race.

A practical guide to follow is to ensure that a runner consumes at least 1.0 g kg^{-1} body weight of carbohydrate each hour over the 4–6 hours immediately post-exercise (Ivy *et al.* 1988b, Blom *et al.* 1987). Following a strenuous exercise session, it is perhaps most palatable to take this carbohydrate in a liquid form. For example, a 65 kg runner would aim to consume approximately 65 g of carbohydrate per hour, or a little over one litre of a 6% (6 g of carbohydrate per 100 ml of fluid) glucose-polymer solution. However, it is important to take on board some solid fuel as soon as possible. In addition to providing the body with energy, this food will also provide raw materials for the repair of damaged tissue and essential nutrients to maintain health and well-being. Popular post-training snacks include jam/banana sandwiches, energy bars, confectionery, breakfast cereals, toast, bananas, raisins and currant buns. This snack should be followed by a further meal based around high-carbohydrate foods (Table 8.4).

THE RUNNER'S REQUIREMENTS OF VITAMINS AND MINERALS

In addition to the *energy providers*, other essential nutrients which must be incorporated into the diet include vitamins and minerals. Vitamins are required in relatively small amounts, but are essential in the regulation of various metabolic processes which ultimately provide the energy to fuel muscle contraction (Van der Beek 1991). There is an argument that runners undertaking high-volume training may require vitamin supplementation due to an increase in vitamin requirements. Assuming that the diet of a runner is equitable in quality to that of an average man or woman, this increase may result from: decreased absorption from the gut; increased excretion in sweat, urine and faeces; or increased turnover as a result of physical exercise (Van der Beek 1991). The scientific literature does not support that the middle or long-distance runner is at risk from vitamin deficiency if their diet conforms to *reference nutrient intakes* (RNIs). There is presently no substantive evidence to support an increased vitamin requirement in runners; moreover vitamin supplementation in runners whose diets meet the RNIs may not further improve performance (Nice *et al*. 1984, Tremblay *et al*. 1984).

There is a linear relationship between energy intake and vitamin intake (Van Erp-Bart *et al*. 1989). Provided a runner's diet is meeting the increased energy demands of their training and that the diet is varied and balanced, the vitamin content of their diet should be well in excess of their needs (Van der Beek 1991). Nevertheless, there is some evidence to support vitamin B complex and vitamin C supplementation to enhance heat acclimatisation (Early and Carlson 1969, Strydhom *et al*. 1976) and vitamins C and E supplementation as antioxidants, especially during periods of intense high-volume training (Chapter 7). Table 8.5 details the principal known water-soluble and fat-soluble vitamins, their potential role in exercise performance and the best food sources in order to meet a recommended level of such vitamins in the diet.

Similar to vitamins, minerals must also be provided in the daily diet. Minerals are involved in a number of functional, structural and regulatory roles. For example, calcium helps to strengthen bone, iron is required in the transport of oxygen to active tissues and magnesium is involved in the regulation of muscle contractions. Refer to Table 8.6 for a more comprehensive description of the roles of the key minerals and their principal dietary sources. Clarkson (1991) suggests that poor diets may be the major cause of mineral deficiencies in athletes, though it is possible that deficiencies in, notably, calcium and iron are exacerbated by strenuous physical training. Calcium supplementation may be prudent in female amenorrhoeic[6] runners in order to promote and maintain healthy bones (Drinkwater *et al*. 1984). Amenorrhoea is associated with lowered

---

[6] Amenorrhoea refers to the absence of a normal menstrual cycle, a condition linked with stress and low percentage body fat. It is a relatively common condition in well-trained female middle and long-distance runners, where failure to menstruate for long periods has been associated with changes in oestrogen secretion and an increased risk of stress fractures.

concentrations of oestrogen, a hormone associated with increased intestinal absorption of calcium, reduced urinary calcium excretion and improved bone mineral density (Lindsay 1987). Thus, female runners may be prescribed supplementary calcium as a precautionary measure against reduced bone mineral density[7].

True iron deficiencies are rare amongst runners, and iron deficiency *per se* does not appear to influence performance. However, iron deficiency anaemia (i.e. a reduction in the amount of haemoglobin in blood, normally associated with an inadequate supply of iron to meet the body's requirements) will have an adverse effect on middle and long-distance running performance. It has been suggested that *sports anaemia* associated with low iron levels in runners may result from the mechanical impact of the foot with the ground (Eichner 1986), though data supporting this observation are equivocal. Nevertheless, runners suffering from an iron deficiency anaemia will experience performance improvements with an appropriate iron supplement. High iron intakes will inhibit zinc absorption; therefore supplements providing around 15 mg day^{-1} are recommended (Clarkson 1991).

Endurance runners involved in intense training may be susceptible to *sports anaemia*, and would therefore benefit from the prudent use of an iron supplement. Vegetarian runners, or those consuming a diet low in meat, also appear to absorb iron from the intestine less efficiently. Caution should always be observed with respect to supplementation, since high iron intakes through inappropriate supplementation are potentially toxic (Department of Health 1991). If you are concerned about your iron status, or indeed your vitamin and mineral status in general, you are advised to consult a general practitioner, or a qualified sports dietician or sports nutritionist.

DIETARY SUPPLEMENTS

As mentioned previously, the need to supplement the diet is only necessary either if there is a dietary deficiency, or if there is a medical condition associated with atypical absorption and/or metabolism. In the case of middle and long-distance runners, if general dietary intake is increased to fuel the increased energy demands of exercise, there will also be commensurate increases in the specific dietary intakes of micro-

---

[7]Reduced bone mineral density is referred to as osteoporosis, and is characterised by a decrease in bone matrix integrity and an increased susceptibility to bone damage.

Table 8.5. Vitamins: functions, dietary sources and recommended nutrient intakes (RNI)

Vitamin	Physiological functions	Dietary sources	Adult RNI
Water-soluble			
Vitamin B complex			
Thiamine (B$_1$)	CHO metabolism; nervous system; muscle growth and muscle tone	Meat, liver, kidney, eggs, whole-grains, cereals, dairy produce, some vegetables and fruit	Women and men 0.4 mg (1000 kcal)$^{-1}$
Riboflavin (B$_2$)	CHO, protein and fat metabolism; cell respiration	Dairy produce, eggs, lean meat, liver	Women: 1.1 mg day^{-1} Men: 1.3 mg day^{-1}
Niacin (B$_3$)	CHO, protein and fat metabolism	Grains, cereals, cheese, fish, eggs, meat, beans, fruit	Women and men 6.6 mg (1000 kcal)$^{-1}$
Pyridoxine (B$_6$)	Protein metabolism; RBC formation	Whole grains, fish, eggs, meat, cereals, leafy vegetables	Women and men 15 μg g^{-1} protein
Cyanocobalamin (B$_{12}$)	CHO, protein and fat metabolism; RBC formation	Meat, fish, dairy produce, eggs, liver	Women and men 1.5 μg day^{-1}
Folic acid (folate)	Regulation of growth; protein breakdown; RBC formation	Green leafy vegetables, legumes, liver, fortified breakfast cereals	Women and men: 200 μg day^{-1}
Biotin	Fat breakdown	Egg yolks, liver, kidney	No RNI
Pantothenic acid	Energy production; fatty acid oxidation	Wide availability in foods	No RNI
Ascorbic acid (C)	Connective tissue; iron absorption/metabolism, healing/infection	Vegetables, fruit, potatoes, fruit and vegetable juices	Women and men: 40 mg day^{-1}

Fat-soluble			
Retinol β-carotene (A)	Growth and repair; connective tissue; skin; vision	Liver, egg, full-fat milk, dark green and orange/yellow vegetables	Women and men: 600 retinol equivalents day^{-1}
Calciferols (D)	Calcium metabolism; bones and teeth	Dairy produce, sunlight, fish oils	No RNI
Vitamin E	Antioxidant; enzyme synthesis and transport	Pure vegetable and nut oils, butter, vegetable spreads, nuts seeds, milk, eggs	0.4 mg α-tocopherol equivalents day^{-1} dietary PUFA
Vitamin K	Blood clotting; fat digestion; glycogen formation	Cereals, vegetables	No RNI

Nutrient data from Paul and Southgate (1978) and Department of Health (1991). Physiological detail from Newsholme and Leech (1983).

Table 8.6. Main minerals: functions, dietary sources and recommended nutrient intakes (RNI)

Mineral	Physiological functions	Dietary sources	Adult RNI
Calcium	Bone/tooth structure; nerve conduction; blood clotting	Milk and products, canned fish, green leafy vegetables, white bread	Women and men: 700 mg day^{-1}
Magnesium	Neuromuscular transmission; bone formation; enzyme reactions	Whole grain cereals, nuts, green leafy vegetables, dairy produce	Women: 270 mg day^{-1} Men: 300 mg day^{-1}
Phosphorus	Bone and tooth formation; energy metabolism	Grains, cereals, meat, milk, green vegetables, most other foods	No RNI
Sodium	Nerve conduction; fluid balance; acid base balance	Salt, cheese, fish, bacon	Women and men: 1600 mg day^{-1}
Potassium	Nerve conduction; fluid balance; acid base balance	Fruit and vegetables juices	Women and men: 3500 mg day^{-1}
Iron	Haemoglobin/myoglobin structure (O_2/CO_2 transport)	Red meat, liver, fortified breakfast cereals, eggs, nuts, dried fruit, bread, green leafy vegetables, whole grains	Women: 14.7 mg day^{-1} Men: 8.7 mg day^{-1}
Zinc	Enzyme synthesis	Meat, unrefined cereals	Women: 7.0 mg day^{-1} Men: 9.5 mg day^{-1}
Selenium	Antioxidant (membranes); electron transfer	Seafood, meat, fish, grains, cereals	Women: 60 μg day^{-1} Men: 75 μg day^{-1}
Chromium	Glucose and insulin metabolism	Meat, whole grains, legumes, fruit	No RNI

Nutrient data from Paul and Southgate (1978) and Department of Health (1991). Physiological detail from Newsholme and Leech (1983).

nutrients. However, in practice, it is sometimes impossible to provide the body with all that it requires through traditional eating conventions, and there will be cases where supplements may prove necessary. For example, following a hard training session or race a runner's appetite may be suppressed. In such instances carbohydrate-rich sports drinks may provide a palatable and convenient *supplement*, aiding the runner's recovery in terms of replenishing the body's carbohydrate reserves. Perhaps one area of confusion surrounds vitamin and mineral supplements, where many athletes subscribe to the adage of *'one is good therefore two must be better'*. It is beyond the scope of this book to enter the great debate surrounding the specific micronutrient requirements of runners, suffice it to say that such a simplistic philosophy is inappropriate and potentially dangerous. As mentioned previously, vitamins and mineral supplements taken in excess of the recommended dose may build up to toxic levels! Nevertheless, there are situations where supplementation may be appropriate from both a health and a performance perspective.

In the previous section, the use of calcium and iron supplements were shown to offer performance benefits to the runner in circumstances where there was previously a deficiency. Other *in vogue* supplements include: creatine to help improve performance during periods of repeated maximal intensity exercise; caffeine, which is popularly referred to as a *fat burner*; glutamine to boost the immune system and ward off possible infections during the winter months of high volume training (Castell, Poortmans and Newsholme 1996); and antioxidants such as vitamin C, vitamin E and selenium, to help combat oxidative tissue damage (Chapter 7).

Creatine

Creatine is found in the typical omnivorous diet in meat and fish; however the levels found in the modern western, urban diet tend to be low. The normal daily intake is less than 1.0 g (Heymsfield *et al.* 1983), whereas the estimated daily requirement is approximately 2.0 g (Walker 1979). The body is able to manufacture creatine from other amino acids in the diet, but this process might prove inadequate for meeting the demands of maximal exercise. Thus supplementation with creatine has been found to elicit ergogenic effects resulting in improved high-intensity exercise performance (Maughan 1995).

There are a number of typical creatine loading programmes available to the runner. Some manufacturers recommend a five-day loading programme, where runners are required to supplement up to 20 g of creatine per day in four doses of 4–5 g. After this initial loading period, runners then transfer to a maintenance programme, supplementing with 2–3 g of creatine per day. Alternatively, similar gains with respect to increases in muscle creatine concentrations have been achieved through supplementing with lower doses (4–5 g day^{-1}) over longer periods. However, the possible consequences of long-term creatine supplementation are still not clear, and excessive protein supplementation of any form should be discouraged for the reasons discussed previously.

Creatine does not improve the maximum force generating capacity of muscle, rather it improves the capacity of muscle to perform repeated bouts of intensive exercise (Greenhaff *et al.* 1993). However, creatine supplementation does not appear to influence the cardiorespiratory or metabolic responses to submaximal exercise (Green *et al.* 1993), nor does it appear to improve endurance performance (Balsom *et al.* 1993).

As noted previously, supplements will only exert a beneficial effect if there is a deficiency. There is evidence that runners involved in regular endurance training will already have elevated muscle stores of creatine, in comparison with sedentary individuals, prior to any supplementation regime. Moreover, the physiological processes whereby a deficiency in creatine would influence exercise capacity are not the principal limitations to middle and long-distance running performance. An exception to this general statement might be the middle-distance runner who incorporates sprint sets into their training programme. Thus, there is presently no sound evidence to support the use of creatine supplementation in improving middle and long-distance racing performance in trained runners. Furthermore, creatine loading is also associated with a weight gain of approximately 1.0–1.5 kg in an average runner, which would potentially be detrimental to performance.

Caffeine

Caffeine is present in the diet as a constituent of many beverages and foods (Table 8.7); nevertheless it is listed as a restricted drug by the International Olympic Committee (IOC). The present IOC legal limit would be a dose resulting in urine caffeine concentrations of less than 12 μg ml^{-1} of urine. The stimulant effects of caffeine may improve high-intensity sprinting exercise performance, but this would require doses greater than the legal limit (Tarnopolsky 1994). With respect to prolonged exercise, caffeine ingestion equivalent to approximately 3–6 mg kg^{-1} body weight (which would result in urine caffeine concentrations below the current IOC limit) has been shown to improve endurance (Costill *et al.* 1977, Costill, Dalsky and Fink 1978). The mechanisms underpinning such performance benefits remain unclear, though some

Table 8.7. Caffeine content of common beverages and foods

	Caffeine (mg per serving)
Coffee (250 ml)	
instant	60–90
drip	75–125
brewed/percolated	95–150
Tea (250 ml)	
weak	40–50
strong	60–75
Cola (375 ml)	40–50
Chocolate (50 g)	10–15

Adapted from Tarnopolsky *et al.* (1994).

possible reasons include: a stimulation of fat metabolism resulting in a sparing of the finite carbohydrate reserves; improved excitation of active muscle; stimulation of the central nervous system; and a decrease in potassium accumulation in blood (where increases in potassium concentrations have been associated with fatigue). The true mechanism is probably a combination of a number of physiological processes, rather than simply a modification of the energy supply–demand relationship as is popularly believed.

The adverse effects of caffeine ingestion as an ergogenic aid are very variable depending upon how much caffeine is ingested per dose and an individual's caffeine tolerance. The generally reported side effects include: insomnia resulting in a decrease in total sleep time and reduced quality of sleep; increased urine production, which may precipitate dehydration and heat stroke if caffeine ingestion precedes prolonged exercise; tremor and symptoms of anxiety and restlessness; and possibly elevated blood pressure in caffeine naive runners (Tarnopolsky 1994). Therefore, if no caffeine is consumed in any form at present, there may be some performance benefits for middle and long-distance runners, though equally any benefits might be offset by deleterious side effects. For runners who are regular caffeine consumers, the doses required to elicit any potentially favourable effects may be in excess of IOC regulations.

Glutamine

Glutamine is an amino acid that performs a number of roles in the body. Importantly for the athlete, one of its most important roles appears to be as a fuel for cells of the immune system (Ardawi and Newsholme 1985). Under resting conditions, tissues in the body such as muscle, lung and brain are net producers of glutamine, whilst others, including cells of the immune system and the gastrointestinal tract, are net users. Under physiologically stressful conditions, such as during and following strenuous training, net producers of glutamine (muscle) may become net users. It has therefore been suggested that as the availability of glutamine is reduced, the function of the immune cells becomes impaired (Parry-Billings *et al.* 1990), and this might in turn be responsible for the high incidence of immunosuppression and ensuing viral infection in endurance athletes (Parry-Billings *et al.* 1992). In addition, tissue damage during intense periods of training or competition (Chapter 7) may further compete for the lowered stores of glutamine, further aggravating the situation. Ingesting an oral glutamine supplement (5 g L-glutamine dissolved in approximately 350 ml of water taken immediately following training or competition) to maintain the body's glutamine balance, has been shown to reduce the incidence of infection in marathon runners (Castell, Poortmans and Newsholme 1996). Nevertheless, it should be noted that as is so often the case in sports nutrition, unequivocal scientific evidence is lagging behind the supplement manufacturers, and we do not know the long-term story of habitual glutamine supplementation.

Bicarbonate, Citrate, Phosphate

With respect to intensive aerobic exercise, such as middle-distance running, fatigue is partly associated with an increase in hydrogen ion concentration in association with lactate accumulation (Sahlin 1992). Supplementation with principally *bicarbonate*, but also *citrate* and *phosphate*, has been suggested as a means of buffering (or counteracting) the effects of hydrogen ion accumulation. The research examining this area of supplementation has yielded very variable results. The consensus appears to be that ingestion of bicarbonate salts in solution, at a dosage of approximately 0.3 g kg^{-1} body weight, may improve performance during repeated sprints or intensive exercise (Horswill 1995). Nevertheless, the potential adverse reactions of some athletes to bicarbonate loading, such as gastrointestinal distress and diarrhoea, suggests that any runners experimenting with this strategy should do so during training in the first instance. Even if a runner experiences performance benefits in training with no ill effects, they would be wise to still demonstrate caution; the anxiety of the competitive situation might further exacerbate any potentially adverse gastrointestinal reactions.

Other Dietary Supplements Claimed to Benefit Middle and Long-Distance Runners

In addition to the more tried and tested nutritional supplements, there are a number of more controversial supplements now on the market. For example, *ginseng, bee pollen* and *Royal jelly* are all marketed as general tonics with a range of alleged therapeutic and restorative benefits that might improve athletic performance. The evidence to support many of the claims made by supplement manufacturers is often limited, or even taken out of context. At the very least, some supplements may simply be a waste of money; however, more worrying is that there are supplements which might actually be harmful if taken unsupervised.

The mineral *chromium* is an essential trace element involved in the release of energy from carbohydrate and fat to fuel exercise. It is therefore marketed on the basis of its fat-burning properties and a claim that it can help improve strength. The body absorbs approximately 3% of dietary chromium, with the remainder being excreted in urine. Diets high in simple sugars and strenuous exercise appear to further increase urinary chromium losses. However, chromium supplementation has not been found to build muscle, increase strength or promote fat metabolism. The protein-like substance *carnitine* has also been advocated as a fat burner. Its principal role in the body is as a carrier in the process by which fatty acids are transported into muscle fibres. It has been argued that carnitine supplementation might promote fatty acid transport and availability in the muscle cell, and would therefore facilitate their subsequent oxidation to fuel exercise. This is a plausible line of reasoning; supplementation will increase blood concentrations of carnitine but this does not result in increases in muscle carnitine concentrations (Hawley, Brouns and Jeukendrup 1998) nor does it appear to alter fat utilisation (Vukovich, Costill and Fink 1994).

Coenzyme Q_{10} (ubiquinone) is a micro-nutrient which plays a role in the series of energy producing chemical reactions which take place in the mitochondria of cells. Supplementation is associated with increases in blood concentrations, but is not associated with increases in muscle concentrations. Thus, coenzyme Q_{10} has not been shown to improve $\dot{V}O_{2max}$ or endurance performance (Braun *et al.* 1991). *Medium-chain triglyceride (MCT) oil* is another nutritional supplement that has been speculated to improve endurance performance. The fatty acids in MCT oil are digested, absorbed and metabolised more readily than normal dietary fats (Bremer and Osmundsen 1984), and are therefore more immediately available to fuel exercise. The potential performance benefits of MCT oils are probably best realised during ultra-endurance races where the exercise intensity will be relatively low. However, ingestion of

MCTs prior to exercise has not been shown to improve endurance performance (Ivy, Costill and Fink 1980, Sabatin *et al.* 1987) and may be associated with gastrointestinal problems if taken in high doses (Hawley, Brouns and Jeukendrup 1998).

KEY POINTS

- The benefits of optimum sports nutrition are not experienced through snatched healthy options just prior to competition, nor can they be obtained by popping the latest nutrient pill, rather they are the result of balanced, habitual eating habits.
- There are seven components to a healthy, well-balanced diet: carbohydrate, fat, protein, vitamins, minerals, fibre and water.
- Carbohydrate, fat and protein are the energy providers of the diet, of which carbohydrate is arguably the most important for the runner.
- The recommended carbohydrate intake for a middle and long-distance runner is equivalent to 8.0–9.0 g kg^{-1} body weight day^{-1}, which would be between 520 and 585 g of carbohydrate per day for a 65 kg runner. This intake might need to be increased to around 10.0 g kg^{-1} body weight day^{-1} (i.e. 650 g day^{-1} in a 65 kg runner) during periods of particularly intense periods of training or competition.
- Dietary protein provides the basic building blocks for tissue growth and repair, and therefore the nature and quality of protein intake should be considered carefully, especially during periods of training; recommended daily intake for the middle or long-distance runner is equivalent to 1.2–1.4 g kg^{-1} body weight day^{-1} (i.e. 78–91 g day^{-1} in the 65 kg runner).
- The fat component of the diet should not make up more than approximately 25% of a runner's total energy intake. However, a fat intake of less than approximately 30 g day^{-1} may compromise the provision of fat-soluble vitamins and essential fatty acids necessary for general good health.
- Vitamins and minerals are only required in relatively small amounts, but are essential for good health and hence ultimately the ability to maintain optimal performance. Therefore vitamins and minerals, in the recommended RNI levels, should be contained within a balanced diet on a daily basis.
- Refuelling during exercise has been shown to benefit race performance during longer (i.e. half-marathon and marathon) distance events. Consuming a 2–8% carbohydrate beverage, which contains a small amount of electrolytes, little and often (e.g. 100–150 ml 10 min^{-1}, or approximately 0.5 l every hour) appears to be the best approach.

- To optimise recovery following training or competition, it is essential to start the refuelling process as soon as possible. Liquid feeds appear to be most palatable immediately post-exercise, providing the equivalent of 1.0 g kg^{-1} body weight h^{-1} (i.e. 65 g h^{-1} in the 65 kg runner) of carbohydrate over the initial 4–6 hours.
- Dietary supplements are generally only necessary if there is a deficiency. Runners should be cautious not to succumb to the advertising claims supporting often expensive nutritional products; there is no such thing as a 'quick fix', neither is there any substitute for quality training.

Chapter 9

Running and the Environment

Joanne L. Fallowfield

INTRODUCTION

Few sporting events take place within the confines of fully air-conditioned venues, where the environment can be carefully controlled between some predefined optimal limits. However, even middle and long-distance races taking place at indoor meetings could be affected by their own micro-environment, which may result in less than ideal running conditions. For the majority of outdoor events, the principal environmental stressors are the low barometric pressure of altitude, temperature, humidity, solar radiation and air quality. This Chapter discusses the influence of the environment on athletic performance and the ways in which the middle or long-distance runner might improve their tolerance and maintain running performance.

RUNNING AT ALTITUDE

Performance in middle and long-distance running is dependent upon the supply of oxygen to the muscle. This, in turn, is dependent upon the pressure gradient which drives the delivery of oxygen from the atmosphere to the mitochondria in muscle; the higher the atmospheric pressure, the greater the oxygen driving force. The physiological challenge of exercising at high altitude results from a decrease in air (barometric) pressure with increases in height above sea level. As barometric pressure falls the oxygen driving force also falls, although the relative percentages of gases in atmospheric air stay approximately the same (i.e. 79.04% nitrogen, 20.93% oxygen, 0.03% carbon dioxide plus trace amounts of other gases).

Thus, as the pressure of oxygen in atmospheric air falls (and hence the availability of oxygen in the runner's lungs), the supply of oxygen to tissue will eventually become compromised. Hypoxia refers to the condition where there is an inadequate supply of oxygen to the tissues in order to meet their needs for energy metabolism. In addition to this physiological limitation, there are a number of other climatic considerations associated with moderate and high-altitude environments which may affect athletic performance. These include extreme atmospheric temperatures (especially with respect to temperature changes between night and day), low humidity, increased intensity of solar radiation due to the thinner air and extreme and sometimes erratic local weather conditions.

The decision of the International Olympic Committee to hold the 1968 Olympic Games in Mexico City (at an altitude of 2300 m above sea level) gave tremendous impetus to research examining the influence of altitude on sporting performance. Subsequent observations from the Games revealed that performances in events of less than 800 m were improved (e.g. 1–2% improvements in events of 100 to 200 m) in the thinner air and lower gravity experienced at this moderate altitude. But performances in events longer than 800 m were progressively impaired (e.g. 5–7% impairments in 3000 m to marathon races) (Noakes 1991).

The general observation of a runner first arriving at altitude is that breathing is perceived as being more difficult. This is despite the actual energy cost of breathing being reduced due to the thinner air and the reduced air pressure on the outer walls of the chest. Almost immediately on arrival at altitude, an athlete will normally start to hyperventilate (i.e. increased frequency of breathing). This will increase the excretion of carbon dioxide from the lungs, resulting in lower acidity (lower pH) of blood. Those athletes who do not demonstrate an initial hyperventilatory response appear to be more susceptible to suffering from the symptoms of acute mountain sickness, a condition that occurs at high altitudes due to altitude hypoxia (characterised by symptoms including shortness of breath, general fatigue, headaches and nausea). Therefore all athletes should be closely monitored over the first few hours following ascent and immediately returned to lower levels if an athlete fails to respond.

Hyperventilation of the thinner, dryer air increases the loss of water from the body through evaporation from the respiratory surfaces of the airways and lungs. This is further exacerbated by evaporation of moisture from the skin. If ignored by not adopting an appropriate drinking strategy to replace lost fluid, such factors will contribute to an increase in the rate of dehydration of the runner resulting in a reduction in plasma volume. This will result in an *apparent* increase in red blood cell and blood haemoglobin concentrations, which might be viewed favourably in terms of the oxygen transport system. The loss in total plasma will also reduce the oxygen and carbon dioxide carrying capacity of blood as a whole. The heart must work harder to pump the thicker, more viscous blood around the body and is therefore placed under increasing stress.

REDUCTION IN $\dot{V}O_{2max}$ AT ALTITUDE

As mentioned previously, the lower barometric pressure of altitude will reduce the oxygen pressure of inspired air, and therefore the oxygen pressure down in the alveolar sacs of the lungs. However, the rate of diffusion of oxygen across the walls of the lung from the alveoli and into blood does not change, and the oxygenation of blood is limited by a reduced pressure gradient. Thus, it might be argued that $\dot{V}O_{2max}$ at altitude is primarily limited by oxygen transport across the lung.

As oxygen moves from the alveoli of the lung and into the pulmonary blood vessels, the reduced driving pressure limits the ability of haemoglobin to 'load-up' with oxygen, and the amount of oxygen transported in arterial blood will be reduced. Similarly at the muscle, the reduced availability of oxygen in blood will limit oxygen delivery to the mitochondria. The body attempts to compensate for this reduced oxygen driving force at the muscle by increasing blood flow from the heart. Thus, heart rate tends to be elevated on initial exposure to altitude.

Maximal oxygen uptake will begin to decrease noticeably from around an altitude of approximately 1500 m. Initially, the rate of reduction is equivalent to approximately 10% for every 1000 m above 1200 m (Squires and Buskirk 1982). However, this rate of decrease in $\dot{V}O_{2max}$ will become greater at higher altitudes; interestingly, well-trained endurance athletes may notice impaired $\dot{V}O_{2max}$ even at altitudes of around 900 m.

A limitation in maximum oxygen uptake arising from incomplete oxygenation of blood in the lung has been termed exercise-induced hypoxaemia and results in a decrease in oxygen transport from the lung to muscle (Chapter 5). Altitude exposure would tend to exacerbate this problem and hence a greater than anticipated decrease in $\dot{V}O_{2max}$ would be experienced by runners susceptible to exercise-induced hypoxaemia (Lawler, Powers and Thompson 1988, Martin and O'Kroy 1992). This may partly explain the large variability in responses to altitude exposure and training amongst endurance athletes, where those limited by cardiac output (i.e. heart limited) may respond better than those who experience exercise-induced hypoxaemia (i.e. lung limited).

INFLUENCE OF ALTITUDE ON DETERMINANTS OF MIDDLE AND LONG-DISTANCE RUNNING PERFORMANCE

As discussed in Chapters 3 and 4, middle and long-distance running performance is not only determined by an athlete's $\dot{V}O_{2max}$, but is also determined by $\%\dot{V}O_{2max}$ sustained, running economy and anaerobic capacity (middle distance runners only). Despite a possible beneficial reduction in the energy cost of breathing at altitude, the absolute oxygen cost of running at race pace will be similar to sea-level. Therefore, as the ability to supply muscle with oxygen and hence $\dot{V}O_{2max}$ are reduced, the muscle oxygen demands remain constant and the runner's relative exercise intensity for the same race pace will increase. To compound the reduction in $\dot{V}O_{2max}$ and the resulting increase in relative exercise intensity, a runner's sustainable $\%\dot{V}O_{2max}$ is also reduced, as reflected in an earlier onset of blood lactate accumulation (OBLA). This sequence of events resulting in earlier fatigue during submaximal running would be evident as a left shift in the OBLA–running speed (exercise intensity) curve (Figure 9.1), which under normal circumstances would be associated with a detraining response.

Anaerobic capacity might also decrease on initial exposure to altitude, as the compensatory hyperventilation response will *blow off* carbon dioxide, and hence reduce the ability of blood to buffer the hydrogen ions

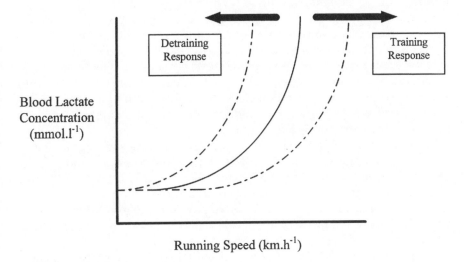

Figure 9.1. Schematic representation of the blood lactate–running speed relationship and the influence of training and detraining

associated with lactate production during intensive exercise. This will be reflected in an increase in muscle and blood lactate concentrations at altitude for the same absolute running speed, resulting in an earlier onset of fatigue.

As well as influencing respiratory and cardiovascular function, altitude hypoxia appears to have a direct effect on muscle function, being associated with a decrease in muscle contractility (i.e. reduced rate of muscle shortening). This is reflected in a loss of muscular power or a loss of *form* in the runner. From a physiological perspective, reduced muscle contractility will be associated with a decline in running economy and an increase in the oxygen cost of maintaining the same absolute running speed.

Thus, from a consideration of respiratory, cardiovascular and muscular responses to altitude hypoxia, the determinants of middle and long-distance running performance, namely $\dot{V}O_{2max}$, % $\dot{V}O_{2max}$ sustained, running economy and anaerobic capacity, are reduced on initial exposure to altitude.

ACCLIMATISATION TO ALTITUDE

It is arguable that if an athlete is involved in a short duration race at altitude (less than 800 m) they may benefit from arriving at the event shortly before competition and leaving soon after. However, for the middle and long-distance runner, competing in a major Games or Championships, this 'quick in-quick out' strategy would not be appropriate. A period of habituation or acclimatisation to altitude, improving a runner's tolerance to the reduced oxygen availability, would be necessary if race performance is to be maintained (Pugh 1967, Levine *et al.* 1990). Alternatively, a runner may feel that the adaptations associated with altitude exposure may be beneficial for subsequent sea-level performances, and would therefore consider incorporating an altitude training camp into their season's preparation.

From a practical perspective, a sea-level middle or long-distance runner travelling to altitude will initially experience around a 15% reduction in $\dot{V}O_{2max}$ (Pugh 1967). This decrease in $\dot{V}O_{2max}$ will impair aerobic performance, where reduced performance will be relative to the increase in altitude and would be greater for longer distance races. Following approximately four week's habituation, this decrease in $\dot{V}O_{2max}$ might be reduced by around 5%. However, it should be noted that any gain in $\dot{V}O_{2max}$ is very individual and will partly reflect a runner's initial tolerance to altitude exposure. If this runner competed immediately on arrival, their performance would normally be impaired.

However, they may not be troubled by some of the other problems resulting from altitude exposure, such as symptoms of mountain sickness or involuntary[1] dehydration if appropriate drinking strategies are not put into place. From a practical perspective, the worst time to compete appears to be between three and six days after arrival, when the body is feeling the full effects of the altitude challenge at a time when it has not really had significant opportunity to begin adapting in order to cope.

It is therefore important, perhaps more so for the longer distance races, that if a runner is to compete at altitude they undergo some kind of altitude habituation or acclimatisation programme prior to the event. The acclimatisation process commences immediately on arrival at altitude, with small, principally biochemical changes taking place in muscle and blood as soon as the body begins to experience the stimulus of reduced oxygen availability (Saltin 1996). Indeed, the initial responses to altitude hypoxia might be viewed as the first steps in a longer term acclimatisation process. However, it will take several weeks before any real functional adaptations are evident that will influence running performance.

Under normal circumstances, where for practical reasons a runner will rarely spend more than six to eight weeks at altitude, there is no evidence that the structure and function of the respiratory system is changed during this relatively short stay. This is in agreement with a view that aerobic performance is not normally limited by the lung (Poole and Richardson 1997). Perhaps the most readily observed acclimatisation physiological adjustments are in the volume and composition of blood. Following the initial dehydration associated with the thinner, dryer air resulting in a decrease in plasma volume, a prolonged stay at altitude is associated with an increase in plasma volume. In addition, the number of red blood cells will also increase (i.e. polycythaemia), along with increases in their volume and their haemoglobin content. Consequently, the capacity of blood to pick up oxygen from the lungs and carry it to tissue is improved. A further modification to blood, namely an increase in 2,3-diphosphoglycerate (2,3-DPG) concentrations in red blood cells (a chemical that reduces the affinity of haemoglobin for oxygen), improves the capacity of blood to *off load* its oxygen on arrival at the capillary bed of tissue.

At the same time as blood is undergoing modification, there are structural changes taking place within the muscle capillary bed. The result of these structural changes is an increase in the density of the capillary network supplying muscle tissue. This was previously thought

---

[1]Involuntary dehydration refers to an unconscious dehydration resulting from an inadequate fluid intake in the face of an increased fluid loss from the body.

to be only due to an opening up of dormant capillaries and a growth of new capillaries over the long term. However, more recently this apparent increase in capillary density has been attributed to a reduction in the cross-sectional size of muscle fibres (Saltin 1996). As the diameters of individual muscle fibres are reduced, the distance between adjacent capillaries will also be reduced, and therefore there will appear to be more capillaries per unit cross-sectional area of whole muscles. From an oxygen delivery perspective, this will improve the capacity of the capillary network to service tissue with the provision of oxygen and nutrients, and the removal of carbon dioxide and waste. However, from a performance perspective, a reduction in muscle fibre size, and hence muscle cross-sectional area, will reduce the force generating capacity of muscle. This, in turn, will have implications for situations where power and acceleration are essential in optimising running performance.

With respect to the structure of individual muscle fibres, altitude exposure is associated with an increase in the myoglobin content of tissue (Wolski, McKenzie and Wenger 1996). The role of myoglobin in muscle is two-fold: first, it facilitates the transport of oxygen from the blood capillaries and into the muscle fibre; and second, especially at the onset of exercise, it can provide muscle with a small, transient store of oxygen. Altitude training has also been associated with an increase in mitochondria number within the muscle fibre. As discussed previously, the mitochondrion is described as the *power house* of the muscle fibre, being the site of aerobic energy metabolism and hence the final destination of the oxygen transported from the atmosphere. Increasing the number of mitochondria will further facilitate the transport of oxygen into the fibre and its subsequent utilisation in the production of energy. However, it has been difficult to discriminate in the scientific studies whether this adaptation is as a result of the training stimulus at altitude, or the hypoxia stimulus *per se* at altitude.

A secondary acclimatisation response is the restoration of normal blood acidity following the hyperventilatory increase in pH. To return blood pH to a normal level of around 7.4, the kidneys excrete the transient excess in bicarbonate ions[2]. However, one consequence of this re-adjustment is a reduction in the body's capacity to manage the hydrogen ions associated with high intensity exercise (i.e. reduced buffering capacity). This will reduce a runner's tolerance to intense exercise, or more specifically a runner's tolerance to the increase in blood

---

[2]Bicarbonate ions represent part of the blood's hydrogen ion buffering capability (along with plasma protein and haemoglobin), being formed from carbon dioxide as a by-product of carbonic acid production.

lactate accumulation and hydrogen ion concentrations. This is reflected in a left shift in the exercise intensity–blood lactate concentration curve normally associated with a detraining response (Figure 9.1). Buffering capacity is restored over time to normal levels, and during a prolonged stay at altitude will eventually be increased (Mizuno *et al.* 1990). Svedenhag *et al.* (1991) followed seven elite middle-distance runners during a two week training camp at altitude (2000 m). During this relatively short stay anaerobic capacity (as measured by MAOD) and muscle buffering capacity increased by approximately 20% and remained elevated relative to pre-altitude exposure levels for at least seven days following return to sea-level. This is an interesting observation as it may explain the benefits reported by sprint/power athletes who incorporate altitude acclimatisation as part of their pre-competition preparations.

ALTITUDE ACCLIMATISATION AND SEA-LEVEL PERFORMANCE

Evidence to support altitude training as part of a runner's pre-season training is currently equivocal. Most of the studies that have shown a positive potentiating effect of altitude acclimatisation on sea-level performance involved volunteers who were not very well trained before travelling to altitude. Consequently, it is difficult to discriminate between the performance improvements due to normal training adaptations of these previously untrained individuals, and those adaptations due to altitude acclimatisation. A further complication in trying to distinguish the benefits, or otherwise, of altitude training is the associated 'camp syndrome' that can either work for or against the runner. For many athletes, training is accommodated into their busy lives along with family, work and social commitments. Thus, an opportunity to spend a period of time focusing exclusively upon training and running performance is a luxury seldom experienced. As a consequence, any performance benefits might simply reflect this exclusivity of attention, resulting in improved quality of training. Alternatively, some athletes can respond adversely to the training camp environment, finding the atmosphere restrictive and claustrophobic, and therefore debilitating with respect to their competition preparations.

The adaptations to altitude exposure are similar and complementary in nature with adaptations to aerobic training (Burtscher *et al.* 1996, Wolski, McKenzie and Wenger 1996). Therefore, there is a rationale for incorporating altitude training into a runner's pre-season conditioning programme. On the negative side, the quality of training in terms of intensive race pace work will be reduced, especially on first arrival, which will be associated with a loss of *sharpness*. From a performance perspective, Noakes (1991) advocates a 'live high–train low' strategy. The potentially favourable physiological adaptations occur in response to habituation to altitude, or living at altitude, rather than training at altitude *per se*. Continuing to train at sea-level, or an altitude that will not adversely impinge upon performance, will help to ensure that the quality of training and race fitness are maintained.

For an altitude training camp to be of any real value to the middle or long-distance runner it would need to be for a minimum of two to six weeks and at an altitude of between 2000 and 3000 m (Dick 1992, Levine and Stray-Gunderson 1992). There appears to be an upper limit of human tolerance to altitude of around 5000 m, beyond which acclimatisation is limited and exercise capacity progressively deteriorates (McFarland 1972).

RUNNING IN THE HEAT: CONTROLLING BODY TEMPERATURE

Thermoregulation refers to the combined physiological processes which regulate body temperature within a relatively narrow range. In a temperate environment and under normal resting conditions, body temperature will rarely fluctuate by more than 1.0°C from an average temperature of 37°C. Effective thermoregulation is largely influenced by a runner's heat acclimatisation status (Wenger 1988), endurance training status (Armstrong and Pandolf 1988), hydration (fluid) status (Sawka and Pandolf 1990) and the type of clothing worn (Gonzalez 1988). Challenges to this thermoregulatory ability include prolonged exercise at moderate to high intensity, illness or infection and changes in local environmental conditions. This section discusses the mechanisms of heat production and heat loss, which normally allow a fine control of body temperature to be achieved.

The hypothalamus is the region in the brain that has been described as the athlete's 'thermostat'. Like the thermostat controlling the central heating in a domestic house, the hypothalamus initiates heat production or heat loss mechanisms with reference to a 'set-point' temperature. Neurones in the preoptic area of the anterior hypothalamus (i.e. central thermoreceptors) monitor the temperature of blood passing through the brain. These receptors are sensitive to changes in blood temperature, such that overheating or excessive cooling of this area in the brain results in the stimulation of appropriate thermoregulatory mechanisms. In addition to these central receptors, there are peripheral thermoreceptors located in the skin to monitor skin and local environmental temperature. The peripheral thermoreceptors similarly relay their message to the hypothalamus, where they are processed and appropriate responses initiated. This central processing also allows voluntary control over continued exposure to the adverse environmental challenge, for example a runner might reduce exercise intensity or move to a cooler environment.

There are four mechanisms by which heat may be lost from the body, and these are conduction, convection, radiation and evaporation. Conductive heat loss involves the transfer of heat from one material (e.g. body core) of a relatively higher temperature, to another (e.g. skin and eventually to the immediate environment) of a relatively lower temperature through direct contact. The body might also gain heat in this way, if the local environment is hotter than skin or deep body temperature (i.e. greater than 37°C).

Convective heat loss involves the transfer of heat from one location to another through the motion of a gas or a liquid. For example, air passing over the skin of a runner will remove heat from its surface. The rate of heat transfer in this way is proportional to the rate of air movement. It therefore follows that a trained runner who is working hard will generate a relatively large amount of additional heat energy, but will also be able to dissipate this heat effectively by virtue of their speed of movement through the air. Therefore, heat loss by convection will be proportional to the running speed sustained for the duration of the race. As with conduction, heat may also be gained by the body through convection, if the environmental temperature is greater than body temperature, independent of the rate of air movement.

The loss of heat through radiation results from the emission of infrared rays. Under resting conditions when the ambient temperature is equivalent to normal room temperature (21–25°C), a runner will lose around 60% of their excess heat through radiation. However, this proportion decreases during prolonged, intense exercise, as other mechanisms of heat dissipation begin to play greater roles. A runner training or racing in direct sunlight may experience radiative heat gain. One strategy to reduce this effect would be to wear loose, light coloured (preferably white) clothing.

The fourth mechanism of heat dissipation is via the evaporation of moisture (sweat) from the skin's surface. Under resting conditions in a relatively temperate environment, there is a continuous insensible loss of fluid from the skin which, when combined with the evaporation of moisture from the respiratory tract, may account for around 30% of the daily fluid loss from the body. During exercise or when the environmental temperature is high, the sweating mechanism is of increasing importance in maintaining a constant core temperature. Indeed, the evaporation of sweat may account for the loss of up to 80% of the body's excess heat production during exercise. An increasing core temperature relative to the hypothalamus' set-point is associated with the initiation of the sweat loss mechanism. Blood flow to peripheral capillaries in the skin is increased. This in turn is associated with an increase in sweat production and sweat secretion from glands in the skin onto the skin's surface. Heat is then drawn from the surrounding area of the body to evaporate the sweat. It is this process of vaporising sweat that results in the loss of heat from the body.

As the body temperature of an exercising runner starts to increase, the hypothalamus will send signals to the smooth muscle which acts as a cuff to regulate blood flow to the skin. The smooth muscle relaxes and peripheral blood flow is increased, facilitating heat loss from the body core. The start of sweat secretion from the sweat glands occurs some 5–10 min following the initiation of exercise (depending upon the training and heat acclimatisation status of the runner). This delay reflects the time lag between starting to exercise and a significant increase in core temperature sufficient to stimulate a thermoregulatory response. In a situation where the runner's core temperature has dropped below the set-point (e.g. when ambient temperature is very low, or during the later stages of long-distance events where the runner is fatiguing and heat dissipation mechanisms out pace the level of heat generation), mechanisms to promote the conservation or production of heat are initiated.

RUNNING IN THE HEAT: THE DUAL CHALLENGE OF EXERCISE

The cardiovascular system of a runner exercising in the heat will face a dual challenge: on the one hand, exercising muscle will require a high blood supply in order to supply oxygen and nutrients, and remove carbon dioxide and waste products; whilst on the other, peripheral blood flow to the skin needs to be increased to facilitate heat loss. If either role is substantially compromised, running performance will be impaired.

As discussed earlier, the sweating mechanism for heat dissipation requires water to be evaporated from the skin's surface. Thus, for sweating to be effective the water vapour pressure (i.e. the water content of atmospheric air) gradient between the runner's skin and the surrounding air must be high. In a hot–dry environment (e.g. during the Desert Marathon of the Sahara), where ambient humidity is low, the runner's sweating response may be switched into over-drive, rapidly losing heat but also dehydrating the runner if fluid intake is not consciously addressed. Conversely, in a hot–wet environment where ambient humidity is high (e.g. in tropical or equatorial regions of the world), the effectiveness of the sweating mechanism in removing heat from the body is reduced as the water vapour pressure gradient between skin and the surrounding air is very small or even non-existent. Thus, the greatest challenge for the runner with respect to the capacity to thermoregulate would be a hot–wet environment, where heat might be gained from the surrounding environment. The sweating mechanism will provide very little in the way of a cooling effect, as sweat would simply drip from the skin.

HEAT ACCLIMATISATION

As with altitude, the body can undergo a degree of physiological adaptation to the environmental challenge of heat and humidity, and tolerance to exercising in the heat is improved. Acclimatisation to heat appears to be much more rapid in comparison with altitude, with the majority of adaptation taking place within the initial 12–14 days of exposure (Pandolf and Young 1992). Though similar to altitude acclimatisation, the degree of heat acclimatisation that takes place is individual to each runner; some runners may never significantly adapt to training and competing in a hot and humid environment. Some of the adaptations discussed later may persist for a number of weeks following heat exposure, though there is a reduction in general heat tolerance three to four days post acclimatisation on returning to temperate conditions. The process of de-acclimatisation is relatively rapid, taking place at a rate of approximately 15–30% per week.

Acclimatisation to the heat (independent of the added thermal stress of high relative humidity) lowers the setting of the hypothalamic set-point (Nadel 1977), so that processes bringing about a cooling of the body are initiated earlier. Exposure to heat without exercising results in only slight acclimatisation responses. Similarly, regular aerobic training in a relatively temperate environment, aside from the desired training effects of the programme, will also be associated with adaptations that will improve a runner's heat tolerance. However, optimal acclimatisation is achieved through exercising (moderate intensity for approximately 60 to 100 min per day) in a heat of 32–35°C (90–95°F) and a relative humidity of greater than 70% (Young, Fricker and Maughan 1998). The intensity and duration of exercise at the start of the acclimatisation period may need to be reduced depending upon the initial training and acclimatisation status of the runner. Thereafter the programme should be progressive, increasing towards optimal levels as quickly as is appropriate for each individual runner. Thus, runners who intend to participate in middle and long-distance events under conditions associated with a high environmental heat stress, should train in the heat for at least one week before the event in order to optimise their performance (Pandolf and Young 1992).

Acclimatisation centres around adaptations to the cardiovascular system, primarily with respect to its role in thermoregulation. Total blood volume is increased through an increase in plasma volume (Senay, Mitchell and Wyndham 1976). This increase in plasma volume (which may be of the order of 12%) is associated with an increase in plasma protein concentrations. Stroke volume (the volume of blood pumped by the heart per beat) is also increased, resulting in a lower resting and submaximal exercise heart rate after approximately seven days of exposure. Cardiac output is maintained as the increased stroke volume accommodates the decrease in heart rate. Venous return to the heart from the systemic circulation is also improved; when linked with the increase in total blood volume, the ability to maintain a stable blood pressure, especially during prolonged exercise, is improved. The net result of these adjustments in cardiovascular functioning is that, relative to initial exposure, core temperature after seven day's exposure is lower at rest and during submaximal exercise. This relative reduction in core temperature, in turn, will help ease the conflict in cardiac output distribution between working muscles and blood flow to the skin. Thus, for the same ambient temperature and humidity, skin temperature at rest and during submaximal exercise is reduced.

An acclimatisation-related increase in plasma volume helps maintain stroke volume, central blood volume (and hence blood pressure) and the ability to dissipate heat through the sweating response. The sweating response also undergoes adaptation following heat exposure. The initiation of the sweating response occurs earlier following heat acclimatisation (Nadel 1977); that is a smaller increase in core temperature will initiate sweat secretion. There is an increase in the actual density of sweat glands per unit area of the skin's surface, which will help to ensure a better distribution of sweat over the skin and therefore further facilitate heat dissipation. In addition, the volume of sweat secreted per gland and per unit time is increased, though from a conservation perspective, the salt concentration (specifically sodium) of sweat is reduced. This is due to the actions of aldosterone, a sodium-conserving hormone released from the adrenal glands. Total sweat production might increase by as much as 100% following full acclimatisation (Leithead and Lind 1964), which will in turn have implications for a runner's drinking strategy in a hot environment if dehydration is not to ensue.

TECHNICAL BOX 9.1

Paradoxical Onset of Shivering with Elevated Core Temperature

During prolonged exercise, even though core temperature is normally elevated, runners may experience a shivering response associated with the appearance of *goose bumps* on the skin's surface. This occurs when dehydration elevates the set-point of the hypothalamus in excess of the already raised core temperature. Thus, the body *believes* itself to be *cold* and initiates an inappropriate cold response. This should be viewed as an early warning sign of impending hyperthermic problems, and the runner should proceed with caution. This *paradoxical hypothermia* can be differentiated from a *real hypothermia* in that the runner will feel excessively hot in the case of the former.

Acclimatisation occurs in response to the elevation of core temperature for a period of time. The key to effective acclimatisation, therefore, is to maintain gentle exercise in the heat, where duration and frequency take precedence over intensity. Acclimatisation sessions should start at an easy pace, where the aim is specifically to raise core temperature and to maintain this elevated temperature over a sustained period of time. Gradually increase the intensity and duration of the training session throughout the acclimatisation period of one to two weeks, taking care not to train too hard ... for too long ... too early. The best advice is to listen to your body, and perhaps to monitor your heart rate response to fairly 'easy' standard sessions if you are accustomed to doing so, and therefore have some typical data for comparison. During acclimatisation and throughout your stay, monitor the hydration status of your body at all times and combine the exercise-acclimatisation programme with an appropriate progressive rehydration strategy (see later). An individual runner's hydration status can be readily monitored either by monitoring body weight (i.e. check weighing every morning and before and after training sessions, where fluid deficits will be reflected in rapid losses in body weight) or by monitoring urine volume and colour (i.e. infrequent urination resulting in a small volume of darkly coloured urine would be associated with dehydration). It is important to remember that fluid needs will increase as your body adapts, and though the body's tolerance of the heat improves, you cannot improve your tolerance of dehydration.

FLUID BALANCE IN THE MIDDLE AND LONG-DISTANCE RUNNER IN THE HEAT

A 60–65 kg runner will normally be carrying around 36–39 litres of fluid in various body compartments. The major routes of water loss during exercise include evaporation from the skin and evaporation from the respiratory tract. Thus, exercise intensities that result in a significant increase in minute ventilation (increased depth and frequency of breathing) will be associated with a relatively high rate of evaporative fluid loss from the respiratory tract. Other avenues of water loss include excretion from the kidneys as a constituent of urine and excretion from the large intestine in faeces. The body would be able to survive for several weeks if it were deprived of food; however it would not survive for more than a few days without water. Furthermore, the previous section has examined mechanisms in which the body may adapt and improve its tolerance to heat, but it cannot be over-emphasised that the body cannot adapt to high levels of water deficiency or dehydration.

Dehydration resulting from inadequate fluid intake, or incomplete rehydration, will impair middle and long-distance running performance (Armstrong, Costill and Fink 1985). Any level of dehydration is potentially limiting to the trained runner; however, the scientific literature suggests that a body weight loss equivalent to 2% dehydration (i.e. equivalent to approximately 1.2–1.3 kg reduction in body weight in a 60–65 kg runner) will significantly impair athletic performance (Armstrong, Costill and Fink 1985). The body can normally tolerate a level of dehydration as great as a 5–7% reduction in body weight, though this is possibly approaching the healthy (or unhealthy) limit. A dehydratory loss in body weight of greater than 7% has been associated with problems in salivating and even swallowing.

TECHNICAL BOX 9.2

Hormonal Regulation of Fluid Balance

As discussed previously, the sweating response draws water from blood plasma. As plasma volume is reduced, the ability of the cardiovascular system to transport oxygen and nutrients to tissue, whilst removing carbon dioxide and waste metabolites, becomes impaired. Thus, following dehydration, tissue oxygen delivery and uptake during intense exercise will be reduced, whilst the exercise heart rate response and associated cardiovascular stress will be increased (Montain *et al.* 1998). The control of fluid balance through hormonal regulation is influenced by changes in both plasma volume and plasma osmolality (a measure of the solute content of plasma). A decrease in plasma volume, usually associated with a commensurate increase in plasma osmolality, stimulates the secretion of renin from the kidneys and anti-diuretic hormone (ADH) from the posterior pituitary gland in the brain. Aldosterone is in turn secreted from the adrenal glands in response to increasing blood concentrations of renin. The action of aldosterone is to promote sodium and water retention in the kidney and hence protect against a decreasing plasma volume. Similarly, ADH promotes water reabsorption in the kidneys, such that plasma volume and central blood pressure are protected.

REHYDRATION IN TEMPERATE AND HOT AND HUMID ENVIRONMENTS

The golden rule for the middle and long-distance runner in a hot and/ or humid environment is to avoid dehydration rather than having to take action to rehydrate. However, in a practical context, a runner will undoubtedly experience some level of dehydration to a greater or lesser extent on a regular basis. Indeed, from observations made in a large number of international athletes from a wide range of sports, it is true to say that a high proportion of athletes are relatively dehydrated, even under resting conditions, in a temperate climate. There are three principal limitations to effective rehydration: gastric emptying or the rate at which fluid passes through the stomach and into the small intestine; intestinal absorption or the rate at which fluid is absorbed from the small intestine into blood; and finally, the retention of this fluid by the body through avoiding or limiting the action of mechanisms associated with urine formation. The last of these three limitations is probably the most significant, as it is often not considered by the athlete who will simply equate drinking, regardless of what is being ingested, with rehydration. The problems with this simplistic view will now be discussed.

The composition of the beverage chosen by the runner has important implications for all three of these potentially limiting processes. Perhaps most importantly the beverage must be palatable (i.e. taste, consistency and serving temperature), otherwise a runner will not drink an appropriate volume in the first instance. The volume, or more specifically the feeding pattern, (i.e. how much and how often), will influence both gastric emptying and intestinal absorption. The best advice is to drink little and often both at rest and where possible during exercise, depending upon personal tolerance to exercising with fluid in the gut. This will ensure that optimal rates of flow are maintained through the gastrointestinal system and facilitate subsequent absorption in the small intestine. It is difficult to give hard and fast advice on drinking patterns, as this will relate both to the nature of the training session, the regulations of a race, as well as any individual preferences of the runner. As a general guide, levels of fluid intake must substantially off-set levels of fluid loss if performance is not to be significantly impaired. Some guidelines on structuring a runner-specific feeding pattern are given in Table 9.1. Other factors concerning beverage formulation that will influence its ability to maintain fluid balance include energy content (which for most purposes will reflect the carbohydrate content of a beverage), osmolality, pH (acidity or alkalinity) and temperature.

A number of practical issues will also inform the formulation of a sports beverage. As well as rehydrating the body, sports drinks are also a convenient way of providing additional energy. However, there is a compromise between energy provision and rehydration The more energy

Table 9.1. Guidelines on structuring individual drinking strategies

1. Estimated fluid loss at rest:	$33 \, ml \, kg^{-1}$ body weight
e.g. 55 kg runner	1815 ml or 1.815 litres
60 kg runner	1980 ml or 1.98 litres
65 kg runner	2145 ml or 2.145 litres

2. Estimated fluid loss during exercise
   Temperate (i.e. 10–20°C) $0.5–1.5 \, l \, h^{-1}$
   Hot (i.e. 25–35°C) $2.0–3.0 \, l \, h^{-1}$
   These figures are estimates based on average data. The absolute rate of fluid loss during exercise will be specific for each runner depending upon their size, intensity of exercise, acclimatisation status and training status
3. Actual fluid loss during training can be estimated by subtracting post-exercise body mass from the sum of pre-exercise body mass and the weight equivalent of the volume of fluid consumed during exercise
   i.e. 1.0 litre of fluid consumed approximately equals 1.0 kg
4. The daily fluid loss will be the sum of the fluid loss at rest and the total fluid loss during exercise. This can be evaluated by check-weighing every morning, and before and after training
5. Estimated total daily fluid replacement
   This will be equivalent to 1.5-times the total estimated fluid loss. This apparent 'excess' is to compensate for any loss of ingested rehydration fluid by the kidneys

in a drink, the slower it will escape the stomach and arrive in the intestine for subsequent absorption, and hence the rate of rehydration will be reduced. Furthermore, a concentrated, energy-rich solution lying in the runner's intestine will draw fluid from the surrounding cells rather than promoting rapid hydration. During hot, or hot and humid conditions, the emphasis for a runner's drinking strategy must be rehydration and hence the drink will contain less energy making it generally more dilute. Conversely, whilst training or competing under cooler ambient conditions, dehydration may be less of a primary concern and the focus of the runner's drinking strategy may shift towards energy provision. Thus, the optimum formulation of a sports drink will be dependent upon local environmental conditions, as well as being influenced by the taste preferences and the associated 'gastrointestinal comfort' of different athletes.

Returning to the problem of simply equating drinking with rehydration and the significance of fluid retention by the body by avoiding or limiting the action of the kidney in urine formation. You will recall that fluid balance is regulated by monitoring changes in plasma volume and plasma osmolality (Technical Box 9.2). This was discussed previously in the context of decreases in plasma volume, possibly associated with increases in plasma osmolality, initiating mechanisms of fluid conservation. In contrast, drinking beverages of large volume and/or low osmolality (e.g. plain water or dilute cordial beverages) will increase plasma volume, decrease plasma osmolality and initiate mechanisms associated with fluid loss. The consequence for the runner might be involuntary dehydration, as the beverage consumed is not being effectively retained by the body. The formulation of sports beverages, specifically their electrolyte (salt) content (especially sodium), acts to oppose the decrease in plasma osmolality in order to promote retention of the fluid by the body. This action of the electrolytes is also facilitated by the carbohydrate content of a beverage. Thus, both the volume and the composition of a beverage are important in maintaining fluid balance.

It is imperative that runners experiment with different beverages and different feeding patterns during training to identify their individual preference. The formulation of the preferred beverage may also be modified depending upon local climatic conditions, and whether the drink is to be taken before, during, or after training or competition. With respect to pre- or post-exercise consumption, the role of a beverage will change from being part of the preparation process (i.e. maintaining hydration, with some energy provision), to being part of the recovery process (i.e. rehydration and replenishing fuel stores). Table 9.2 provides some practical advice to consider when choosing the optimum sports drink formulation.

Table 9.2. Guidelines for an optimum 'Sports' beverage

Factor		Recommendation
Palatability	Taste	All athletes have their personal preference, though it should be remembered that as the athlete exercises and core temperature increases, so the perception of taste changes Strong flavours may not be appropriate
	Temperature	$\sim 9–10°C$
	Consistency	'Light' drinks rather than 'thick' drinks; sticky, simple glucose drinks can become nauseous
	Carbonation	Still is preferable during exercise; 'gassy' drinks are associated with excess 'wind'
Carbohydrate	Type	Glucose polymers (e.g. maltodextrins)
	Concentration	$\sim 6–8\%$* (where % equates to $g(100\ ml)^{-1}$)
Electrolytes	Type	Sodium is the most important Specific electrolyte content will vary; however chloride, potassium and magnesium are relatively common
	Concentration	Varies with carbohydrate content to maintain optimal osmolality. Most important is sodium: $20–25\ mmol\ l^{-1}$
Osmolality		Optimal: $\sim 300\ mosmol\ kg^{-1}$ Influenced by carbohydrate and electrolyte content
Volume	Feeding pattern	'Little and often' Depending upon the circumstances, an initial drink of $\sim 200–300$ ml, followed by ~ 100 ml at least every 10–15 min

* The actual percentage carbohydrate content will vary depending upon whether the drink is for rehydration (2% CHO) or energy replenishment (11% CHO), and this will influence osmolality.

PRE-COOLING AS A STRATEGY FOR REDUCING OR DELAYING BODY TEMPERATURE INCREASES WHILST EXERCISING IN THE HEAT

The negative effects of hot, or hot and humid environments on running performance appear to be associated with increases in body (core) temperature. Thus, any strategy that would reduce, or delay, this increase in body temperature might hold some benefit for improving middle or long-distance running performance under these conditions. Pre-event cooling was one strategy that was first reported in the scientific literature in the early 1980s (Schmidt and Bruck 1981), but did not gain significant popular interest until the mid-1990s prior to the 1996 Olympic Games in Atlanta, USA.

The physiological rationale for pre-cooling is based upon a lowering of skin temperature, and hence establishing a greater temperature gradient for dissipating heat from *deeper* regions of the body (Schmidt and Bruck 1981). Furthermore, cooler skin temperatures might also be associated with a smaller proportion of the total cardiac output being directed towards the skin and therefore possibly allowing a greater volume of blood to be directed to contracting muscle. From the previous discussion, lower skin and body temperature will also delay the onset of sweating and decrease the sweating rate, thus conserving body fluid during endurance events (Hessermer *et al.* 1984). Strategies involving a 30 min exposure to cold air (Lee and Haymes 1995) or 20 min exposure to cold water (Booth, Marino and Ward 1997), have been associated with improved running performance in moderate (i.e. 24°C) and hot (i.e. 32°C) environments. Such pre-cooling approaches, whilst resulting in some performance benefits, would not really be practical for the pre-race preparations of the middle and long-distance runner. A more contemporary approach would therefore be to use cooling jackets or strategically positioned ice packs.

Research from the Australian Institute of Sport prior to the Atlanta Games demonstrated that the use of cooling 'ice' jackets, worn during warm-up and/or during competition, reduced the rate of increase in core temperature and lowered sweating rates during subsequent exercise. However, the success of pre-cooling appeared to be dependent upon limiting the intensity and duration of any warm-up so that core temperature was not elevated prior to competition; the wearing of a cool jacket allowed athletes to perform competition-specific exercise intensities during warm-up without substantially elevating core temperature. Thus, pre-cooling by way of an ice jacket may hold some benefit for a middle or long-distance runner when competing in hot, or hot and humid environments.

RUNNING IN THE COLD

The human body is less able to cope with cold than it is with heat. Generally, behavioural changes (e.g. wearing additional clothing and taking shelter) protect ourselves from cold exposure. Indeed, physiological mechanisms for conserving body temperature and generating additional heat are considerably less effective in comparison with the mechanisms of heat dissipation. Mechanisms of heat conservation and/or heat production are initiated when blood temperature falls below the set-point of the hypothalamus. The relatively immediate coping mechanisms include: skeletal muscle shivering; non-shivering thermogenesis (i.e. heat production through a sympathetic nervous response increasing energy metabolism in cells); and peripheral vaso-constriction (i.e. a decrease in blood flow to skin). Over the longer term the body's innate insulation might be increased through laying down more fat. Factors influencing a runner's ability to conserve body heat include: body composition (i.e. fat content of the body versus lean muscle mass); body size (i.e. the ratio of surface area to volume); and possibly training status.

In terms of cold stress, the rate of temperature reduction is propor-tional to both the duration of exposure and the temperature gradient between the body and its immediate environment. Hypothermia is the condition characterised by an abnormally low body temperature (less than 35°C) and is associated with a rapid deterioration in physical and mental performance. If core temperature drops below approximately 32°C, the mechanisms of heat production become inadequate, and such cold exposure will soon become life threatening. A runner exposed to cold on a regular basis will notice a small degree of acclimatisation; for example, skin temperature at the onset of shivering and the amount of shivering are both reduced (Davies and Johnston 1961).

In terms of running performance, the physiological responses to cold exposure will effect the respiratory system, the cardiovascular system, energy metabolism and muscle function. A reduction in core temperature is associated with a decrease in $\dot{V}O_{2max}$ (Bergh and Ekblom 1979b), whilst the rate of oxygen uptake is increased both at rest and during submax-imal exercise (i.e. decreased running economy). These transient changes in response to cold exposure would be experienced by the runner as being analogous to a general detraining effect. Consequently, as perform-ance during middle and long-distance running is in part determined by $\dot{V}O_{2max}$ and running economy, race times will increase in proportion to the reduction in core temperature.

In addition, impaired contractility of heart muscle following cold exposure is associated with a reduced maximal heart rate and a commensurate decrease in maximal cardiac output (Rennie *et al.* 1980). At rest and during low-intensity exercise, central blood pressure is maintained through vasoconstriction of skin capillaries, which whilst promoting an increase in venous return, also improves the insulatory capacity of the body. A reduction in blood temperature associated with a decline in core temperature reduces the amount of oxygen unloaded from blood to tissue as it passes through muscle capillaries. This may contribute to the reduction in $\dot{V}O_{2max}$. However, with in-creasing exercise intensity, shivering is suppressed and muscle de-mand for blood flow over-rides the cold-induced vasoconstriction (Toner and McArdle 1988). Metabolic heat production in well-trained runners during exercise will help defend body temperature. Tissue oxygen delivery is therefore maintained so that $\dot{V}O_{2max}$ may not be compromised.

Independent of any exercise effects, cold exposure leading to a reduction in core temperature will stimulate an increase in metabolic rate in order to increase heat production (Nadel *et al.* 1973). The additive effect of this increased metabolic rate during exercise is that a runner will require a greater rate of energy turnover in order to run at the same absolute speed (i.e. relative exercise intensity is increased). In addition, any reduction in muscle blood flow associated with cooling (Rennie *et al.* 1980) will increase the rate of anaerobic energy production resulting in an increase in lactate (and hydrogen ion) formation. This sequence of events would result in an earlier onset of fatigue during submaximal running in association with a depletion of the body's limited carbohydrate stores, evident as a left shift in the lactate–running speed curve (Figure 9.1).

Aside from these cardiovascular and metabolic adjustments, the velocity and power of muscle contraction are reduced through cold exposure (Bergh and Ekblom 1979a) and the pattern of muscle fibre recruitment is changed. A consequence of this is that running economy will be further impaired as muscle efficiency is reduced. Thus, from a performance perspective, it is evident that cold exposure associated with a decrease in core temperature will result in decreases in the determinants of middle and long-distance running performance.

AIR QUALITY AND PERFORMANCE

Poor air quality or air pollution is an increasing problem for the modern-day athlete, not just from a health perspective, but also from the link between poor air quality and impaired exercise performance (Pandolf 1988). The potential adverse effects of air pollution are dependent upon: the type of pollutant; its particular size; how readily it can dissolve in water; effects on pulmonary function; and concentration relative to dose–response characteristics (Table 9.3) (Pierson *et al.* 1986).

The principal action sites of air borne pollutants are the lungs (influencing mechanical function and oxygen diffusion) and the cardiovascular system (influencing oxygen transport). Ozone, sulphur dioxide and nitrogen dioxide impair lung function and irritate the lining of the lungs, such that ventilatory efficiency is impaired. Carbon monoxide, on the other hand, interferes with the transport of oxygen in blood to muscle tissue through competition with oxygen to bind with haemoglobin. The most common pollutant, suspended particles such as pollen or

Table 9.3. Air pollutants and exercise performance

Air pollutant	Upper limit for health	Action
Carbon monoxide	9 ppm	Greater affinity for Hb than O_2 → impairs O_2 delivery to muscle
Carbon dioxide	–	Hyperventilation, headaches, disturbance of ABB
Ozone	0.12 ppm	Decreased lung function, headaches
Sulphuric acid	–	Irritates upper respiratory tract
Sulphur dioxide	0.14 ppm	Increased exercise-induced bronchospasm
Nitrogen dioxide	–	Lung irritant
Suspended particles	150 μg m^{-3}	Aggravation of asthma and obstructive lung disease

ppm = parts per million.
ABB = acid base balance.
Adapted from Robergs and Roberts (1997).

small particles of dirt, will effect those runners who have presented symptoms of a respiratory problem. The extent to which such particles are carried in the air will partly be dependent upon local environmental conditions such as temperature, humidity and air movement. Consequently, the problems of pollution are generally exacerbated during the summer months, when the warmer ambient conditions favour enhanced air borne pollutants.

INTERACTION BETWEEN AIR QUALITY AND AIR TEMPERATURE

The combined stress of extremes in temperature, humidity and air quality will impair submaximal and maximal exercise performance (Pandolf and Young 1992). Photochemical reactions of air borne pollutants, which are carried more easily in warm air, with ultraviolet radiation from the sun result in increased levels of the toxic gas ozone. The environmental consequences of this potentially lethal cocktail are evident in the summer smogs that tend to engulf industrial cities. The tissue-damaging effects of ozone on the respiratory tract are discussed in Chapter 7. However, from a functional perspective, high ambient levels of ozone are associated with an increase in breathing frequency and a decrease in the ventilatory tidal volume (i.e. breathing becomes more shallow). The consequences of these respiratory adjustments will be a reduction in the efficiency of ventilation, and therefore a decrease in the extraction of oxygen from inspired air. If the levels of ozone are high, a runner's $\dot{V}O_{2max}$ and $\%\dot{V}O_{2max}$ sustained will be reduced and hence race times will be increased.

The situation will not necessarily be better for runners during the cooler winter months. For example, the interaction of air borne pollutants and cold air may be responsible for increases in exercise-induced asthma in runners with relatively sensitive airways. The resulting constriction of the airways would limit ventilation (i.e. decreasing $\dot{V}O_{2max}$ and $\%\dot{V}O_{2max}$ sustained), therefore impairing middle and long-distance running performance.

KEY POINTS

- The principal environmental stressors that will impact upon outdoor middle and long-distance running performance can be described in terms of altitude, temperature, humidity, solar radiation, and air pollution.
- The decrease in barometric pressure at altitude reduces the *driving force* of oxygen from the atmosphere, via the lung, to muscle tissue.
- Thus, $\dot{V}O_{2max}$ is reduced at altitude, and running performance is further compromised by reductions in $\%\dot{V}O_{2max}$ sustained, running economy and anaerobic capacity.
- Hyperventilation represents an important initial response on arrival at altitude. Athletes who do not hyperventilate appear to be more prone to suffering from *acute mountain sickness*.
- Runners intending to compete at altitude, or who chose to incorporate altitude acclimatisation as part of their pre-season preparations, may benefit from adopting a 'live high–train low' strategy. This allows the desired physiological adaptations to take place whilst training quality is maintained.
- Running in the heat presents a dual challenge to the cardiovascular system, as exercising muscle and skin (to facilitate heat loss) compete for the available blood supply.
- A runner should allow 12–14 days for their body to adapt significantly to the heat, where acclimatisation is facilitated by combining heat exposure with 60–100 min day^{-1} of moderate intensity exercise. Take care not to exercise too hard ... for too long ... too early!
- The major concern of the runner in a hot, or hot and humid environment is the maintenance of fluid balance. The golden rule should be to avoid dehydration by drinking little and often rather than having to take steps to rehydrate.

- Running performance in the cold is impaired due to decreases in $\dot{V}O_{2max}$ and running economy. A small amount of acclimatisation to the cold is possible, but runners are better advised to dress appropriately.
- Poor air quality will directly impair performance by decreasing $\dot{V}O_{2max}$ and %$\dot{V}O_{2max}$ sustained. The situation is further exacerbated by extremes of temperature and humidity.

Appendix

Peggy Wellington

MEAL PLANS

Tables A.1–A.4 outline the varying nutrient (carbohydrate—CHO, protein and fat) profiles of different meals and snacks. They can all be used as part of a varied programme. These plans are designed to act as a guideline only as their specific composition will vary slightly from different brands of ingredients, and from country to country.

Tables A.3 and A.4 detail only the savoury element of the meal. The addition of a dessert (fruits/yoghurts/buns, etc.) and drinks will boost the carbohydrate content further, as well as improving the overall nutrient profile (assuming the dessert and drink are relatively healthy options). Small quantities of pure vegetable oils should be used in the cooking and preparation of food where relevant in order to provide vitamin E and essential fatty acids.

Table A.1. Nutrient profiles of breakfasts

Breakfasts	CHO (g)	Protein (g)	Fat (g)
Breakfast 1 (386 kcal/1625 kJ)			
50 g bowl fortified wholegrain cereal (e.g. Branflakes)			
250 ml semi-skimmed milk			
small handful of dried fruit (50 g)			
125 ml glass of unsweetened orange juice			
Nutrient information	75	15	5
Breakfast 2 (625 kcal/2625 kJ)			
50 g bowl fortified sweetened cereal (e.g. Frosties)			
250 ml semi-skimmed milk			
2 medium slices of wholegrain toast (80 g)			
scraping of butter (10 g)			
1 small banana (120)			
Nutrient information	100	18	15
Breakfast 3 (700 kcal/2940 kJ)			
4 Scotch Pancakes			
1 large mashed banana			
2 tablespoons of syrup			
250 ml semi-skimmed milk			
Nutrient information	125	17	18
Breakfast 4 (840 kcal/3528 kJ)			
large bowl of porridge (made with whole milk)			
1 tablespoon sugar (25 g)			
1 handful of raisins (50 g)			
250 ml glass of unsweetened orange juice			
1 pear			
Nutrient information	150	23	21
Breakfast 5 (1000 kcal/4200 kJ)			
2 bagels (200 g)			
scraping of butter (10 g)			
3 large tablespoons of baked beans (300 g)			
250 ml glass of unsweetened orange juice			
Nutrient information	175	35	16

Table A.2. Nutrient profiles of different snacks

Snacks	CHO (g)	Protein (g)	Fat (g)
Snack 1 (230 kcal/995 kJ)			
8 dried apricots (150 g)			
Nutrient information	50	6	1
Snack 2 (530 kcal/2270 kJ)			
1 medium slice of fresh fruit cake (150 g)			
Nutrient information	50	5	13
Snack 3 (300–350 kcal/1260–1470 kJ)			
1 bowl cereal (50 g)			
250 ml semi-skimmed milk			
Nutrient information	50	10–15	5
Snack 4 (180 kcal/755 kJ)			
1 large bowl of tinned fruit in syrup (3000 g)			
Nutrient information	50	1	0
Snack 5 (200 kcal/845 kJ)			
1 handful raisins (75 g)			
Nutrient information	50	2	0
Snack 6 (287 kcal/1204 kJ)			
1 Mars bar (65 g)			
Nutrient information	50	4	12
Snack 7 (334 kcal/1412 kJ)			
1 banana sandwich (2 medium slices white bread—80 g)			
scraping of butter (10 g)			
Nutrient information	60	7	10
Snack 8 (415 kcal/1767 kJ)			
Milkshake with:			
250 ml semi-skimmed milk			
1 banana			
150 g carton fruit yoghurt			
1 tablespoon honey (25 g)			
Nutrient information	80	16	5
Snack 9 (714 kcal/3006 kJ)			
Peanut butter and jam on toast with:			
2 thick brown slices of toast (100 g)			
2 tablespoons of peanut butter			
2 tablespoons of jam			
Nutrient information	100	22	30

Table A.3. Nutrient profiles of different light meals

Light meals	CHO (g)	Protein (g)	Fat (g)
Light meal 1 (640 kcal/2550 kJ)			
pasta/rice salad with:			
100 g (dry weight) pasta/rice			
1 diced grilled chicken breast (150 g) or 300 g			
beans (if vegetarian)			
mixture of salad and vegetables			
1 tablespoon oil-based dressing			
Nutrient information	80	60	13
Light meal 2 (760 kcal/3200 kJ)			
scrambled eggs and tomatoes on toast with:			
4 medium slices of brown toast (160 g)			
2 eggs, scrambled			
2 tomatoes			
Nutrient information	100	30	30
Light meal 3 (812 kcal/3438 kJ)			
stuffed rolls with soup:			
2 large wholegrain baps (150 g)			
4 slices (100 g) lean meat			
scraping of butter (10 g)			
lots of salad			
1 can vegetable soup (400 g)			
Nutrient information	120	53	17
Light meal 4 (690 kcal/2915 kJ)			
jacket potato with beans and cheese:			
1 large jacket potato (250 g)			
3 tablespoons of baked beans (300 g)			
25 g of hard cheese			
Nutrient information	125	30	10
Light meal 5 (880 kcal/3751 kJ)			
tuna and butter bean salad with pitta bread:			
canned tuna (100 g or half a can)			
1 can butter beans (or any beans, 400 g)			
150 g tomatoes			
1 teaspoon olive oil			
2 pitta breads			
Nutrient information	150	60	10

Table A.4. Nutrient profiles of different main meals

Main meals	CHO (g)	Protein (g)	Fat (g)
Main meal 1 (873 kcal/3667 kJ)			
Spaghetti Bolognese and vegetables with:			
100 g/medium handful (dry weight) spaghetti			
300 g/3 large tablespoons of Bolognese			
50 g/2 tablespoons peas			
50 g/2 tablespoons sweetcorn			
Nutrient information	100	40	36
Main meal 2 (500 kcal/2120 kJ)			
boiled potatoes and bean and vegetable casserole:			
450 g/9 boiled potatoes			
300 g/3 large tablespoons of casserole			
lots of vegetables			
Nutrient information	100	16	4
Main meal 3 (613 kcal/2590 kJ)			
baked sweet potato and lasagne:			
250 g/large sweet potato			
400 g Lasagne—large portion			
lots of vegetables			
Nutrient information	100	20	13
Main meal 4 (960 kcal/4071 kJ)			
pasta/rice meal and sauce:			
150 g (dry weight) pasta/rice (6–8 tablespoons)			
1 piece lean meat or fish (150 g)			
low fat sauce (200 g or half a jar) such as sweet & sour/BBQ/tomato-based/mesquite/chilli/black bean/napolitana			
lots of vegetables			
Nutrient information	140	72	18
Main meal 5 (708 kcal/3010 kJ)			
vegetable chilli and rice:			
rice (dry weight) 100 g or 4 tablespoons			
vegetable chilli with beans (300 g or 3 large tablespoons)			
lots of vegetables			
Nutrient information	150	28	6

Supplementary Reading

Further texts complementing and extending the information presented in *Improving Sports Performance in Middle and Long-Distance Running* include:

Cavanagh P. R. (ed) (1990) *Biomechanics of Distance Running*. Human Kinetics: Champaign, USA.
Clark N. (1997) *Nancy Clark's Sports Nutrition Guidebook* (2nd edition). Human Kinetics: Champaign, USA.
Daniels J. (1998) *Daniels' Running Formula*. Human Kinetics: Champaign, USA.
Greene L., Pate R. (1997) *Training for Young Distance Runners*. Human Kinetics: Champaign, USA.
Martin D. E., Coe P. N. (1997) *Better Training for Distance Runners*. Human Kinetics: Champaign, USA.
Newsholme E., Leech T., Duester G. (1994) *Keep on Running*. John Wiley and Sons: Chichester, UK.
Noakes T. (1991) *Lore of Running*. Human Kinetics: Champaign, USA.
Williams M. H. (1998) *The Ergogenics Edge*. Human Kinetics: Champaign, USA.

References

Alessio H. M., Goldfarb A. H. (1988) Lipid peroxidation and scavenger enzymes during exercise: adaptive response to training. *Journal of Applied Physiology*, **64**: 1333–1336.

Allen W. K., Seals D. R., Hurley B. F., Ehsani A. A., Hagberg J. M. (1985) Lactate threshold and distance-running performance in young and older endurance athletes. *Journal of Applied Physiology*, **58**: 1281–1284.

Amiel D., Akeson W. H., Harwood F. L., Frank, C. B. (1983) Stress deprivation effect on metabolic turnover of the medial collateral ligament collagen. *Clinical Orthopaedics and Related Research*, **172**: 265–270.

Andersen P., Henriksson J. (1977) Training induced changes in some groups of human type II skeletal muscle fibres. *Acta Physiologica Scandanavica*, **99**: 123–125.

Anderson T. (1996) Biomechanics and running economy. *Sports Medicine*, **22**: 76–89.

Ardawi M. S. M., Newsholme E. A. (1985) Metabolism in lymphocytes and its importance in the immune response. *Essays in Biochemistry*, **21**: 1–44.

Armstrong L. E., Costill D. L., Fink W. J. (1985) Influence of diuretic-induced dehydration on competitive running performance. *Medicine and Science in Sports and Exercise*, **17**: 456–461.

Armstrong L. E., Pandolf K. B. (1988) Physical training cardiorespiratory physical fitness and extreme-heat tolerance. In: Pandolf K. B., Sawka R. R., Gonzalez R. R. (eds), *Human Performance Physiology and Environmental Medicine at Terrestrial Extremes*. Benchmark Press: Indianapolis, USA.

Åstrand P.-O. (1967) Diet and athletic performance. *Federation Proceedings*, **26**: 1772–1777.

Bailey S. P., Pate R. R. (1991) Feasibility of improving running economy. *Sports Medicine*, **12**: 228–236.

Bale J., Sang J. (1996) Kenyan Running: Movement, Culture, Geography and Global Change. Frank Cass: London, UK.

Balsom P. D., Harridge S. D. R., Soderlund K., Sjodin B., Ekblom B. (1993) Creatine supplementation *per se* does not enhance endurance exercise performance. *Acta Physiologica Scandanavica*, **149**: 521–523.

Bangsbo J. (1996) Oxygen deficit: a measure of the anaerobic energy production during intense exercise? *Revue Canadienne de Physiologie Appliquee/Canadian Journal of Applied Physiology*, **21**: 350–363.

Bangsbo J., Michalsik L., Petersen A. (1993) Accumulated O_2 deficit during intense exercise and muscle characteristics of elite athletes. *International Journal of Sports Medicine*, **14**: 207–213.

Bendich A. (1991) Exercise and free radicals: Effects of antioxidant vitamins. In: Brouns F. (ed.), *Advances in Nutrition and Top Sport. Medicine and Sport Science*, Karger: Basel, **32**, pp. 59–78.

Bergh U., Ekblom B. (1979a) Influence of muscle temperature on maximal muscle strength and power output in human skeletal muscles. *Acta Physiology Scandanavia*, **107**: 33–37.

Bergh U., Ekblom B. (1979b) Physical performance and peak aerobic power at different body temperatures. *Journal of Applied Physiology*, **46**: 885–889.

Bergstrom J., Hermansen L., Saltin B. (1967) Diet, muscle glycogen, and physical performance. *Acta Physiologia Scandanavia*, **71**: 140–150.

Bilanin J. E., Blanchard M., Russek-Cohen E. (1989) Lower vertebral bone density in male long distance runners. *Medicine and Science in Sport Exercise*, **21**: 66–70.

Billat L. V., Koralsztein J. P. (1996) Significance of the velocity at $\dot{V}O_{2max}$ and time to exhaustion at this velocity. *Sports Medicine*, **22**(2): 90–108.

Blom P. C. S., Hostmark A. T., Vaage O., Vardal K. R., Maehlum S. (1987) Effect of different post-exercise sugar diets on the rate of muscle glycogen resynthesis. *Medicine and Science in Sports Exercise*, **19**: 491–496.

Boileau R. A., Mayhew J. L., Riner W. F., Lussier L. (1982) Physiological characteristics of elite middle and long distance runners. *Canadian Journal of Applied Sport Sciences*, **7**: 167–172.

Booth J., Marino F., Ward J. J. (1997) Improved running performance in hot humid conditions following whole body pre-cooling. *Medicine and Science in Sports and Exercise*, **29**: 943–949.

Bosco C., Montanari G., Ribacchi R. (1987) Relationship between the efficiency of muscular work during jumping and the energetics of running. *European Journal of Applied Physiology*, **56**: 138–143.

Bouchard C. (1990) Discussion: heredity, fitness, and health. In: Bouchard C., Shepard R. J., Stephens T., Sutton J. R., McPherson B. D. (eds), *Exercise, Fitness and Health*. Human Kinetics: Champaign, IL, USA.

Bovens A. M., Janssen G. M., Vermeer H. G., Hoeberigs J. H., Janssen M. P., Verstappen F. T. (1989) Occurrence of running injuries in adults following a supervised training program. *International Journal of Sports Medicine*, **10** (Suppl. 3): S186–S190.

Braun B., Clarkson P. M., Freedson P. S., Kohl R. L. (1991) The effect of coenzyme Q_{10} supplementation in trained cyclists. *International Journal of Sport Nutrition*, **1**: 353–365.

Brouns F., Saris W. H., Rehrer N. J. (1987) Abdominal complaints and gastrointestinal function during long-lasting exercise. *International Journal of Sports Medicine*, **8**: 175–189.

Brown K. M., Morrice P. C., Duthie G. G. (1997) Erythrocyte vitamin E and plasma ascorbate concentrations in relation to erythrocyte peroxidation in smokers and nonsmokers: dose response to vitamin E supplementation. *American Journal of Clinical Nutrition*, **65**: 496–502.

Bremer J., Osmundsen H. (1984) Fatty acid oxidation and its regulation. In: Numa S. (ed.), *Fatty Acid Metabolism and its Regulation*. Elsevier: Amsterdam, pp. 113–154.

Buckle P. M. (1965) Exertional (march) haemoglobinuria. Reduction in hemolytic episodes by use of sorbo–rubber insoles in shoes. *Lancet*, **1**: 1136–1138.

Budgett R. (1990) Overtraining syndrome. *British Journal of Sports Medicine*, **24**: 231–236.

Burtscher M., Nachbauer W., Baumgartl P., Philadelphy M. (1996) Benefits of training at moderate altitude versus sea level training in amateur runners. *European Journal of Applied Physiology*, **74**: 558–563.

Carter D. R. (1984) Mechanical loading histories and cortical bone remodeling. *Calcif. Tissue Int.*, **36**(Suppl. 1): S19–S24.

Casey A., Short A. H., Curtis S., Greenhaff P. L. (1996) The effect of glycogen availability on power output and the metabolic responses to repeated bouts of maximal isokinetic exercise in man. *European Journal of Applied Physiology*, **72**: 249–255.

Castell L. M., Poortmans J. R., Newsholme E. A. (1996) Does glutamine have a role in reducing infections in athletes? *European Journal of Applied Physiology*, **73**: 488–490.

Cavagna G. A., Komarek L., Mazzolein S. (1971) The mechanics of sprint running. *Journal of Applied Physiology*, **217**: 709–721.

Cavanagh P. R., Kram R. (1985) Mechanical and muscular factors affecting the efficiency of human movement. *Medicine and Science in Sports and Exercise*, **17**: 326–331.

Child R. B., Brown S. J., Day S., Donnelly A., Roper H., Saxton J. (1999) Changes in indices of antioxidant status, lipid peroxidation and inflammation in human skeletal muscle after eccentric muscle actions. *Clinical Science*, **96**: 105–115.

Child R. B., Wilkinson D. M., Fallowfield J. (in press) Effects of a 7 day training taper on simulated half–marathon running performance, indices of muscle damage, lipid peroxidation and serum antioxidant protection.

Chilibeck P. D., Sale D. G., Webber C. E. (1995) Exercise and bone mineral density. *Sports Medicine*, **12**: 103–122.

Clarkson P. M. (1991) Minerals: Exercise performance and supplementation in athletes. *Journal of Sports Science*, **9**(Special Issue): 91–116.

Coggan A. R., Spina R. J., Rogers M. A., King D. S., Brown M., Nemeth P. M. and Holloszy J. O. (1990) Histochemical and enzymatic characteristics of skeletal muscle in master athletes. *Journal of Applied Physiology*, **68**: 1896–1901.

Coggan A. R., Williams B. C. (1995) Metabolic adaptations to endurance training: Substrate metabolism during exercise. In: Hargreaves M. (ed.), *Exercise Metabolism*. Human Kinetics: Champaign, IL, USA, pp. 177–210.

Conley D. L., Krahenbuhl G. S. (1980) Running economy and distance running performance in highly trained athletes. *Medicine and Science in Sports and Exercise*, **12**: 357–360.

Conley D. L., Krahenbuhl G. S., Burkett L. N., Millar A. L. (1981) Physiological correlates of female road racing performance. *Research Quarterly for Exercise and Sport*, **52**: 441–448.

Conley D. L., Krahenbuhl G. S., Burkett L. N., Millar A. L. (1984) Following Steve Scott: physiological changes accompanying training. *The Physician and Sportsmedicine*, **12**: 103–106.

Costill D. L. (1972) Physiology of marathon running. *Journal of the American Medical Association*, **221**: 1024–1029.

Costill D. L. (1986) *Inside Running: Basics of Sports Physiology*. Benchmark Press: Indianapolis, USA.

Costill D. L. (1988) Carbohydrates for exercise: dietary demands for optimal performance. *International Journal of Sports Medicine*, **9**: 1–18.

Costill D. L., Bowers R., Branam G., Sparks K. (1971a) Muscle glycogen utilization during prolonged exercise on successive days. *Journal of Applied Physiology*, **31**: 834–838.

Costill D. L., Branam G., Eddy D., Sparks K. (1971b) Determinants of marathon running success. *Internationale Zeitschrift für angewandte Physiologie einschleisslich Arbeitsphysiologie*, **29**: 249–254.

Costill D. L., Coyle E. F., Dalsky G., Evans W., Fink W., Hoopes D. (1977) Effects of elevated plasma FFA and insulin on muscle glycogen usage during exercise. *Journal of Applied Physiology*, **43**: 695–699.

Costill D. L., Dalsky G. P., Fink W. J. (1978) Effects of caffeine ingestion on metabolism and exercise performance. *Medicine and Science in Sports and Exercise*, **10**: 155–158.

Costill D. L., Fink W. J., Pollock M. L. (1976) Muscle fibre composition and enzyme activities of elite distance runners. *Medicine and Science in Sports and Exercise*, **8**: 96–100.

Costill D. L., King D. S., Thomas R., Hargreaves M. (1985) Effects of reduced training on muscular power in swimmers. *The Physician and Sportsmedicine*, **13**: 94–101.

Costill D. L., Miller J. M. (1980) Nutrition for endurance sport: Carbohydrate, and fluid balance. *International Journal of Sports Medicine*, **1**: 2–14.

Costill D. L., Sherman W. M., Fink W. J., Maresh C., Witten M., Miller J. M. (1981) The role of dietary carbohydrates in muscle glycogen resynthesis after strenuous running. *American Journal of Clinical Nutrition*, **35**: 1831–1836.

Costill D. L., Thomason H., Roberts E. (1973) Fractional utilization of the aerobic capacity during distance running. *Medicine and Science in Sports and Exercise*, **5**: 248–252.

Coyle E. F. (1991) Timing and method of increased carbohydrate intake to cops with heavy training, competition and recovery. *Journal of Sports Sciences*, **9**(Suppl.): S29–S52.

Coyle E. F., Coggan A. R., Hopper M. K., Walters T. J. (1988) Determinants of endurance in well-trained cyclists. *Journal of Applied Physiology*, **64**: 2622–2630.

Coyle E. F., Feltner M. E., Kautz S. A., Hamilton M. T., Montain S. J., Baylor A. M., Abraham L. D. and Petrek G. W. (1991) Physiological and biomechanical factors associated with elite endurance cycling performance. *Medicine and Science in Sports and Exercise*, **23**: 93–107.

Craig F. N., Cummings E. G. (1966) Dehydration and muscular work. *Journal of Applied Physiology*, **21**: 670–674.

Cross C. E., Motchnik P. A., Bruener B. A., Jones D. A., Kaur H., Ames, B. N., Halliwell B. (1992) Oxidative damage to plasma constituents by ozone. *FEBS Letters*, **298**: 269–272.

Daniels J. (1974) Running with Jim Ryun: a five year study. *The Physician and Sportsmedicine*, **2**: 63–67.

Daniels J., Daniels N. (1992) Running economy of elite male and elite female runners. *Medicine and Science in Sports and Exercise*, **24**: 483–489.

Daniels J., Oldridge N., Nagle F., White B. (1978a) Differences and changes on $\dot{V}O_2$ among young runners 10 to 18 years of age. *Medicine and Science in Sports and Exercise*, **10**: 200–203.

Daniels J. T., Yarbough C., Foster C. (1978b) Changes in $\dot{V}O_{2max}$ and running performance with training. *European Journal of Applied Physiology*, **39**: 249–254.

Davies C. T. M. (1980) Effects of wind assistance and resistance on the forward motion of a runner. *Journal of Applied Physiology*, **48**: 702–709.

Davies C. T. M., Thompson M. W. (1979) Aerobic performance of female marathon and male ultramarathon athletes. *European Journal of Applied Physiology*, **41**: 233–245.

Davies K. J. A., Quintanilha A. T., Brooks G. A., Packer L. (1982) Free radicals and tissue damage produced by exercise. *Biochemical Biophysiological Research Communications*, **107**: 1198–1205.

Davies T. R. A., Johnston D. R. (1961) Seasonal acclimatization to cold in man. *Journal of Applied Physiology*, **16**: 231–234.

Dempsey J. (1987) Exercise-induced imperfections in pulmonary gas exchange. *Canadian Journal of Applied Sport Sciences*, **12**: 66s–70s.

Department of Health (1991) *Dietary Reference Values for Food, Energy, and Nutrients for the United Kingdom.* HMSO: London, UK.

Dick F. W. (1992) Training at altitude in practice. *International Journal of Sports Medicine*, **13**(Suppl. 1): S203–S209.

Diplock A. T., Charleux J.-L., Crozier-Willi G., Kok F. J., Rice-Evans C., Roberfroid M., Stahl W., Vina-Ribes J. (1998) Functional food science and defence against reactive oxygen species. *British Journal of Nutrition*, **80** (Suppl. 1): S77–S112.

Di Prampero P. E. (1986) The energy cost of human locomotion on land and in water. *International Journal of Sports Medicine*, **7**: 55–72.

Draper S., Wood D., Fallowfield J. L. (1998) Comparison of three protocols for the assessment of maximal oxygen uptake in runners (abstract). *Proceedings of Third Annual Congress of The European College Of Sport Science*, Manchester, p. 271.

Drinkwater B. L., Nilson K., Chestnutt C. H., Bremner W. J., Shainholtz S., Southworth M. B. (1984) Bone mineral content of amenorrheic athletes. *New England Journal of Medicine*, **311**: 277–281.

Dugan M. E., McBurney M. I. (1995) Luminal glutamine perfusion alters endotoxin–related changes in ileal permeability of the piglet. *Journal of Parenteral and Enteral Nutrition*, **19**: 83–87.

Early R. G., Carlson B. R. (1969) Water-soluble vitamin therapy on the delay of fatigue from physical activity in hot climatic conditions. *Int. Zeit. Ang. Physiol.*, **27**: 43–50.

Eichner E. R. (1986) The anemias of athletes. *Physics of Sportsmedicine*, **14**: 122–130.

Elstner E. F., Osswald W. (1991) Air Pollution: Involovement of Oxygen Radicals (a mini review). *Free Radical Research Communications*, **12–13**: 795–807.

Fallowfield J. L., Williams C. (1993) Carbohydrate intake and recovery from prolonged exercise. *International Journal of Sports Nutrition*, **3**: 150–164.

Fallowfield J. L., Williams C., Booth J., Choo B. H., Growns S. (1996) Effect of water ingestion on endurance capacity during prolonged running. *Journal of Sports Science*, **14**: 497–502.

Farrell, P. A., Wilmore, J. H., Coyle, E. F., Billing J. E. and Costill D. L. (1979) Plasma lactate accumulation and distance running performance. *Medicine and Science in Sports and Exercise*, **11**: (4) 338–344.

Fielding R. A., Manfredi T. J., Ding W., Fiatarone M. A., Evans W. J., Cannon J. G. (1993) Acute phase response in exercise III. Neutrophil and IL–1*b* accumulation in skeletal muscle. *American Journal of Physiology*, **265**: R166–R172.

Fisher R., McMahon L. F., Ryan M. J., Larson D., Brand M. (1986) Gastrointestinal bleeding in competitive runners. *Digestive Diseases and Sciences*, **31**: 1226–1228.

Frankel H. (1978) Editorial comments. Stress fractures. *American Journal of Sports Medicine*, **6**: 396.

Fry A. C., Kraemer W. J. (1997) Resistance exercise overtraining and overreaching. Neuroendocrine responses. *Sports Medicine*, **23**: 106–129.

Fry R. W., Morton A. R., Keast D. (1992) Periodisation of training stress—A review. *Canadian Journal of Sports Science*, **17**: 234–240.

Fry R. W., Morton A. R., Keast D. (1991) Overtraining in athletes: an update. *Sports Medicine*, **12**: 32–65.

Fujita T., Sakurai K. (1995) Efficacy of glutamine-enriched enteral nutrition in an experimental model of mucosal ulerative colitis. *British Journal of Surgery*, **82**: 749–751.

Gaesser G. A., Poole D. C. (1996). The slow component of oxygen uptake kinetics in humans In: Holloszy J. O. (ed.), *Exercise and Sports Science Reviews*. Williams and Wilkins: Baltimore, USA.

Gambetta V. (1993) Chinese record breakers – give credit where it is due. *New Studies in Athletics*, **8**(4): 21–22.

Gaudin C., Zerath E., Guezennec C. Y. (1990) Gastric lesions secondary to long distance running. *Digestive Diseases and Sciences*, **35**: 1239–1243.

Gauduel Y., Menasche P., Duvellroy M. (1989) Enzyme release and mitochondrial activity in reoxygenated cardiac muscle: relationship with oxygen-induced lipid peroxidation. *General Physiology of Biophysiology*, **8**: 327–340.

George K. P., Wolfe L. A., Burggraf G. W. (1991) The 'athletic heart syndrome'. A critical review. *Sports Medicine*, **11**: 300–331.

Glaze W. H. (1986) Reaction products of ozone: a review. *Environmental Health Perspective*, **69**: 151–155.

Gledhill N., Cox D., Jamnik R. (1994) Endurance athletes' stroke volume does not plateau; major advantage in diastolic function. *Medicine and Science in Sports and Exercise*, **26**: 1116–1121.

Gohil K., Rothfuss L., Lang J., Packer L. (1987) Effect of exercise training on tissue vitamin E and ubiquinone content. *Journal of Applied Physiology*, **63**: 1638–1641.

Gonzalez R. R. (1988) Biophysics of heat transfer and clothing considerations. In: Panndolf K. B., Sawka M. N., Gonzalez R. R. (eds), *Human Performance Physiology and Environmental Medicine at Terestrial Extremes*. Benchmark Press: Indianapolis, USA, pp. 45–95.

Green A. L., Greenhaff P. L., Macdonald I. A., Bell D., Holliman D., Stroud M. A. (1993) The influence of oral creatine supplementation on metabolism during submaximal incremental treadmill exercise. *Proc. Nutr. Soc.*, **53**: 84A.

Green S. (1990) The relationships between blood-borne and gas-exchange descriptors of anaerobic capacity and short distance running performances. MSc Thesis, University of Victoria, Canada.

Green S., Dawson B. (1993) Measurement of anaerobic capacities in humans: Definitions, limitations and unsolved problems. *Sports Medicine*, **15**: 312–327.

Greenhaff P. L., Casey A., Short A. H., Harris R. C., Soderlund K., Hultman E. (1993) Influence of oral creatine supplementation on muscle torque during repeated bouts of maximal voluntary exercise in man. *Clinical Science*, **84**: 565–571.

Grimston S. K., Tanguay K. E., Gundberg C. M., Hanley D. A. (1993) The calciotropic hormone response to changes in serum calcium during exercise in female long distance runners. *Journal of Clinical Endocrinology and Metabolism*, **76**: 867–872.

Guezennec C. (1995) Oxidation rates, complex carbohydrates and exercise. *Sports Medicine*, **19**: 365–372.

Guttman A. (1978) From ritual to record: the nature of modern sports. Columbia University Press; New York, USA.

Halliwell B., Chirico S. (1993) Lipid peroxidation: its mechanism measurement and significance. *American Journal of Clinical Nutrition*, **57**(Suppl.): 715S–725S.

Halvorsen F.-A., Ritland S. (1992) Gastrointestinal problems related to endurance event training. *Sports Medicine*, **14**: 157–163.

Hargreaves M., Dillo P., Angus D., Febbraio M. (1996) Effect of fluid ingestion on muscle metabolism during prolonged exercise. *Journal of Applied Physiology*, **80**(1): 363–366.

Harris R. C., Edwards R. H. T., Hultman E., Nordesjo L.-O., Nylind B., Sahlin K. (1976) The time course of phosphocreatine resynthesis during recovery of the quadriceps muscle in man. *Pflugers Archive*, **376**: 137–142.

Hawley J. A., Brouns F., Jeukendrup A. (1998) Strategies to enhance fat utilisation during exercise. *Sports Medicine*, **25**: 241–257.

Hesserner V, Langusch D., Bruck K., Bodecker R. H., Breidenbauch T. (1984) Effect of slightly lowered body temperatures on endurance performance in humans. *Journal of Applied Physiology*, **57**: 1731–1737.

Heymsfield S. B., Arteaga C., McManus C., Smith J., Moffitt S. (1983) Measurement of muscle mass in humans. *American Journal of Clinical Nutrition*, **39**: 478–494.

Higuchi M., Cartier L. J., Chen M., Holloszy J. O. (1985) Superoxide dismutase and catalase in skeletal muscle: Adaptive response to exercise. *Journal of Gerontology*, **40**: 281–286.

Hikida R. S., Staron R. S., Hagerman F. C., Sherman W. M., Costill D. L. (1983) Muscle fiber necrosis associated with human marathon runners. *Journal of the Neurological Sciences*, **59**: 185–203.

Horswill C. A. (1995) Effects of bicarbonate, citrate, and phosphate loading on performance. *International Journal of Sports Nutrition*, **5**(Suppl.): S111–S119.

Houmard J. A., Costill D. L., Mitchell J. B., Park S. H., Hickner R. C., Roemmich J. N. (1990) Reduced training maintains performance in distance runners. *International Journal of Sports Medicine*, **11**: 46–52.

Houmard J. A., Scott B. K., Justice C. C., Chenier T. C. (1994) The effects of a taper on performance in distance runners. *Medicine and Science in Sports and exercise*, **26**(5): 624–631.

Howald H. (1982) Training-induced morphological and functional changes in skeletal muscle. *International Journal of Sports Medicine*, **3**: 1–12.

Hunter A. L., Grimble R. F. (1997) Dietary sulphur amino acid adequacy influences glutathione synthesis and glutathione-dependent enzymes during the inflammatory response to endotoxin and tumour necrosis factor–a in rats. *Clinical Science*, **92**: 297–305.

Ivy J. L., Costill D. L., Fink W. (1980) Contribution of medium and long chain triglyceride intake to energy metabolism during prolonged exercise. *International Journal of Sports Medicine*, **1**: 15–20.

Ivy J. L., Katz A. L., Cutler C. L., Sherman W. M., Coyle E. F. (1988a) Muscle glycogen synthesis after exercise: effect on time of carbohydrate ingestion. *Journal of Applied Physiology*, **65**: 1480–1485.

Ivy J. L., Lee M. C., Brozinick J. T., Reed M. J. (1988b) Muscle glycogen storage after different amounts of carbohydrate ingestion. *Journal of Applied Physiology*, **65**: 2018–2023.

Ivy J. L., Withers R. T., Van Handel P. J., Elger D. H. and Costill D. L. (1980)

Muscle respiratory capacity and fibre type as determinants of the lactate threshold. *Journal of Applied Physiology,* **48**: 523–527.

Jackson M. J., Edwards R. H. T, Symons M. C. R. (1985) Electron spin resonance studies of intact mammalian skeletal muscle. *Biochemica Biophysica Acta,* **847**: 185–190.

Jackson M. J., McArdle A., O'Farrel S. (1995) Free radicals, muscle fatigue and damage. In Blake D., Wingard P. G. (ed) *Immunopharmacology of Free Radical Species.* Academic Press, London, pp. 175–182.

James, S. L., Bates B. T., Osternig L. R. (1978) Injuries to runners. *American Journal of Sports Medicine,* **6**: 40–50.

Janssen G. M. E., ten Hoor, F. (1989) Introduction, in Marathon running: functional changes in male and female subjects during training and contests. *International Journal of Sports Medicine,* **10**(Suppl.): S118–123.

Jenkins D. J. A., Thomas D. M., Wolever M. S., Taylor R. H., Barker H., Fielden H., Baldwin J. M., Bowling A. C., Newman H. C., Jenkins A. L., Goff D. V. (1981) Glycemic index of foods: a physiological basis for carbohydrate exchange. *American Journal of Clinical Nutrition,* **34**: 362–366.

Jones A. M. (1998) A five year physiological case study of an Olympic runner. *British Journal of Sports Medicine,* **32**: 39–43.

Karlsson J., Saltin B. (1971) Diet, muscle glycogen, and endurance performance. *Journal of Applied Physiology,* **31**: 203–206.

Kasravi F. B., Adawi D., Molin G., Bengmark S., Jeppsson B. (1996) Dynamics of bacterial translocation in acute liver injury induced by D-galactosamine in rat. *APMIS,* **104**: 135–140.

Keul J., Doll E., Koppler E. (1972) *Energy Metabolism in Human Muscle.* Karger, Basel, Switzerland.

Klausen K., Andersen L. B., Pelle I. (1981) Adaptive changes in work capacity, skeletal muscle capillarisation and enzyme levels during training and detraining. *Acta Physiologica Scandanavica,* **113**: 9–16.

Knight D. R., Schaffartzik W., Poole D. C., Hogan M. C., Bebout D. E., Wagner P. D. (1993) Effect of hyperoxia on maximal leg O_2 supply and utilization in man. *Journal of Applied Physiology,* **75**: 2586–2594.

Kobayashi Y. (1974) Effect of vitamin E on aerobic work performance in man during acute exposure to hypoxic hypoxia. Unpublished Thesis, University of New Mexico.

Kraft R., Ruchti C., Burkhardt A., Cottier H. (1992) Pathogenic principles in the development of gut-derived infectious-toxic shock (GITS) and multiple organ failure. *Current Studies in Hematology and Blood Transfusion,* **59**: 204–240.

Krahenbuhl G. S., Williams T. J. (1992) Running economy: changes with age during childhood and adolescence. *Medicine and Science in Sports and Exercise,* **24**: 462–466.

Krahenbuhl G. S., Morgan D. W., Pangrazi R. P. (1989) Longitudinal changes in distance-running performance of young males. *International Journal of Sports Medicine,* **10**: 92–96.

Kuipers H., Janssen G. M., Bosman F., Frederik P. M., Geurten P. (1989) Structural and ultrastructural changes in skeletal muscle associated with long-distance training and running. *International Journal of Sports Medicine,* **10**(Suppl. 3): S156–S159.

Kyle C. R. (1979) Reduction of wind resistance and power output of racing cyclists and runners travelling in groups. *Ergonomics,* **22**: 387–397.

Lambert E. V., Speechly D. P., Dennis S. C., Noakes T. D. (1994) Enhanced endurance in trained cyclists during moderate intensity exercise following 2 weeks adaptation to a high fat diet. *European Journal of Applied Physiology*, **69**: 287–293.

Lapachet R. A. B., Miller W. C., Arnall D. A. (1996) Body fat and exercise endurance in trained rats adapted to a high-fat and/or high–carbohydrate diet. *Journal of Applied Physiology*, **80**: 1173–1179.

Lawler J., Powers S., Thompson D. (1988) Linear relationship between maximal oxygen uptake and $\dot{V}O_{2max}$ decrement during exposure to acute hypoxia. *Journal of Applied Physiology*, **64**: 1486–1492.

Lee D. T., Haynes E. M. (1995) Exercise duration and thermoregulation responses following whole body precooling. *Journal of Applied Physiology*, **79**: 1971–1976.

Lehmann M., Baur S., Netzer N., Gastmann U. (1997) Monitoring high intensity endurance training using neuromuscular excitability to recognize overtraining. *European Journal of Applied Physiology*, **76**: 187–191.

Lehmann M., Foster C., Keul J. (1993) Overtraining in endurance athletes: a brief review. *Medicine and Science in Sports and Exercise*, **25**(7): 854–862.

Leithead C. S., Lind A. G. (1964) *Heat Stress and Heat Disorders*. Caswell and Co. London, UK. pp. 16–30.

Lemon P. W. R. (1991) Effect of exercise on protein requirements. *Journal of Sports Science*, **9**(Suppl.): 53–70.

Levine B. D., Engfred K., Friedman D. B., Kjaer K., Saltin B. (1990) High altitude endurance training: effect on aerobic capacity and work performance. *Medicine and Science in Sports and Exercise*, **22**(Abstract): S35.

Levine B. D., Stray-Gunderson J. (1992) A practical approach to altitude training: where to live and train for optimal performance. *International Journal of Sports Medicine*, **13**(Suppl. 1): S209–S212.

Lindsay R. (1987) Estrogens and Osteoporosis. *Physiology of Sportsmedicine*, **15**: 91–108.

Londeree B. R. (1986) The use of laboratory test results with long distance runners. *Sports Medicine*, **3**: 201–213.

Mader A., Liesen H., Heck H., Philippi H., Schurch P. M., Hollmann W. (1976) Zur beurteilung der sportartspezifischen audaurleistunsfahigkeit im labor. *Spotartz Sportmed*, **4**: 80–88, **5**: 109–112.

Mair P., Mair J., Bleier J., Waldenberger F., Antretter H., Balogh D., Puschendorf B. (1995) Reperfusion after cardioplegic cardiac arrest – effects on intracoronary leucocyte elastase release and oxygen free radical mediated lipid peroxidation *Acta Anaesthesiologica Scandinavica*, **39**: 960–964.

Maron M. B., Horvath S. M., Wilkerson J. E., Gliner J. A. (1976) Oxygen uptake measurements during competitive marathon running. *Journal of Applied Physiology*, **40**: 836–838.

Maron M. B., Wagner J. A., Horvath S. M. (1977) Thermoregulatory responses during competitive marathon running. *Journal of Applied Physiology*, **42**: 909–914.

Martin D., O'Kroy J. (1992) Effects of acute hypoxia on $\dot{V}O_{2max}$ of trained and untrained subjects. *Journal of Sports Sciences*, **11**: 37–42.

Martin D., Powers S. K., Cicale M., Collop N., Huang D., Criswell D. (1992) Validity of pulse oximetry during exercise in elite endurance athletes. *Journal of Applied Physiology*, **72**: 455–458.

Martin D. E. (1993) Distance running in 1993 – A new standard of excellence. *New Studies in Athletics*, **8**(4): 53–59.

Martin D. E., Coe P. N. (1997) *Better Training For Distance Runners*. Human Kinetics: Champaign, IL, USA.

Martin D. T., Scifres J. C., Zimmerman S. D., Wilkinson J. G. (1994) Effects of interval training and a taper on cycling performance and isokinetic leg strength. *International Journal of Sports Medicine*, **15**: 485–491.

Martin R. B., Burr D. B. (1982) A hypothetical mechanism for the stimulation of osteonal remodelling by fatigue damage. *Journal of Biomechanics*, **15**: 137–139.

Maughan R. J. (1991) Fluid and electrolyte loss and replacement during exercise. *Journal of Sports Science*, **9**(Special Issue): 117–142.

Maughan R. J. (1995) Creatine supplementation and exercise performance. *International Journal of Sports Nutrition*, **5**: 94–101.

Maughan R. J., Leiper J. B. (1983) Aerobic capacity and fractional utilisation of aerobic capacity in elite and non-elite male and female marathon runners. *European Journal of Applied Physiology*, **52**: 80–87.

McCabe M. E., Peura D. A., Kadakia S. C., Bocek Z., Johnston L. F. (1986) Gastrointestinal blood loss associated with running a marathon. *Digestive Diseases and Sciences*, **31**: 1229–1232.

McConell G. K., Costill D. L., Widrick J. J., Hickey M. S., Tanaka H., Gastin P. B. (1993) Reduced training volume and intensity maintain aerobic capacity but not performance in distance runners. *International Journal of Sports Medicine*, **14**: 33–37.

McCord J. M. (1985) Oxygen–derived free radicals in postischemic tissue injury. *New England Journal of Medicine*, **312**: 159–163.

McFarland R. A. (1972) Psychophysiological implications of life at altitude and including the role of oxygen in the process of aging. In: Yousef M. K., Horvarif S. M., Bullard R. W. (eds.), *Physiological Adaptations Desert And Mountain* Academic Press: New York, USA.

McMahon L. F., Ryan M. J., Larson D., Fisher R. L. (1984) Occult gastrointestinal blood loss in marathon runners. *Annals of Internal Medicine*, **100**: 846–847.

Medbo J. I. (1996) Is the maximal accumulated oxygen deficit an adequate measure of the anaerobic capacity? *Canadian Journal of Applied Physiology*, **21**: 370–383.

Medbo J. I., Burgers S. (1990) Effect of training on the anaerobic capacity. *Medicine and Science in Sports and Exercise*, **22**: 501–507.

Medbo J. I., Mohn A.-C., Tabata I., Bahr R., Vaage O., Sejersted O. U. (1988) Anaerobic capacity determined by maximal accumulated O_2 deficit. *Journal of Applied Physiology*, **64**: 50–60.

Medbo J. I., Tabata I. (1989) Relative importance of aerobic and anaerobic energy release during short-lasting exhausting bicycle exercise. *Journal of Applied Physiology*, **67**: 1881–1886.

Medoff R. J. (1987) Soft tissue healing. *Annals of Sports Medicine*, **3**: 67–70.

Messier S. P., Cirillo K. J. (1989) The effects of a verbal and visual feedback system on running technique, perceived exertion and running economy in female novice runners. *Journal of Sports Sciences*, **7**: 113–126.

Miller B. J., Pate R. R., Burgess W. (1988) Foot impact force and intravascular hemolysis during distance running. *International Journal of Sports Medicine*, **9**: 56–60.

Mizuno M., Juel C., Bro-Rasmussen T., Mygind E., Schibye R., Rasmussen B., Saltin B. (1990) Limb skeletal muscle adaptation in athletes after training at altitude. *Journal of Applied Physiology*, **68**(2): 496–502.

Montain S. J., Sawka M. N., Latzka W. A., Valeri C. R. (1998) Thermal and cardiovascular strain from hypohydration: influence of exercise intensity. *International Journal of Sports Medicine*, **19**: 87–91.

Morgan D. W., Baldini F. D., Martin P. E., Kohrt W. M. (1989) Ten kilometer performance and predicted velocity at $\dot{V}O_{2max}$ among well-trained male runners. *Medicine and Science in Sports and Exercise*, **21**: 78–83.

Morgan D. W., Craib M. (1992) Physiological aspects of running economy. *Medicine and Science in Sports and Exercise*, **24**: 456–461.

Morgan D. W., Daniels J. T. (1994) Relationship between $\dot{V}O_{2max}$ and the aerobic demand of running in elite distance runners. *International Journal of Sports Medicine*, **15**: 426–429.

Morgan W. P., Brown D. R., Raglin J. S., O'Connor P. J., Ellickson K. A. (1987) Physiological monitoring of overtraining and staleness. *British Journal of Sports Medicine*, **21**: 107–114.

Morton A. R. (1992) Special medical considerations: asthma In: Bloomfield J., Fricker P. A., Fitch K. D. (eds), *Textbook of Science and Medicine in Sport*. Blackwell Scientific Publications: Melbourne.

Muoio D. M., Leddy J. J., Horvarth P. J., Awad A. B., Pendergast D. R. (1994) Effect of dietary fat on metabolic adjustments to maximal $\dot{V}O_2$ and endurance in runners. *Medicine and Science in Sports and Exercise*, **26**: 81–88.

Mustafa M. G. (1990) Biochemical basis of ozone toxicity. *Free Radical Biology and Medicine*, **9**: 245–265.

Nadel E. R. (ed.) (1977) *Problems with Temperature Regulation During Exercise*, Academic Press: New York, USA.

Nadel E. R., Holmer I., Bergh U., Åstrand P.-O., Stolwijk J. A. J. (1973) Thermoregulatory shivering during exercise. *Life Science*, **13**: 983–989.

Newsholme E. A., Leech A. R. (1983) *Biochemistry for the Medical Sciences*. John Wiley & Sons: Chichester, UK.

Nice C., Reeves A. G., Brinck-Johnson T., Noll W. (1984) The effect of pantothenic acid on human exercise capacity. *Journal of Sports Medicine and Physical Fitness*, **24**: 26–29.

Noakes T. D., Myburgh K. H., Schall R. (1990) Peak treadmill running velocity during the $\dot{V}O_{2max}$ test predicts running performance. *Journal of Sports Sciences*, **8**(1): 35–45.

Noakes T. D. (1991) *Lore of Running*. Human Kinetics: Champaign, IL, USA.

Noyes F. R., DeLucas J. L., Torvik P. J. (1974) Biomechanics of anterior cruciate ligament failure: an analysis of strain-rate sensitivity and mechanisms of failure in primates. *Journal of Bone Joint Surgery*, **56-A**: 236–253.

Noyes F. R., Torvik P. J., Hyde W. B., DeLucas J. L. (1974) Biomechanics of ligamaent failure. II. An analysis of immobilisation, exercise, and reconditioning effects in primates. *Journal of Bone Joint Surgery*, **56-A**: 1406–1418.

Ogawa S. (1970) Effect of vitamin E and vitamin C compound on aerobic physical performance in cold environment. *Republic of Sports Science Research of Japanese Amateur Sports Association*.

Packer L. (1997) Oxidants, antioxidant nutrients and the athlete. *Journal of Sports Sciences*, **15**: 353–363.

Pandolf K. B. (1988) Air quality and human performance in Pandolf K. B., Sanka M. N., Gonzalez R. (Eds) Human Performance Physiology and Environmental Medicine at Terrestrial Extremes. Benchmark Press Inc. Indianapolis: 591–629.

Pandolf K. B., Young A. J. (1992) Environmental extremes and endurance performance. In: Shephard R. J., Åstrand P.-O. (eds), *Endurance in Sport*. Blackwell Scientific Publishing: Oxford, UK, pp. 270–282.

Parry-Billings M., Evans J., Calder P. C., Newsholme E. A. (1990) Does glutamine contribute to immunosuppression? *Lancet*, **336**: 523–525.

Parry-Billings M., Budgett R., Koutedakis Y., Blomstrand E., Brooks S., Williams C., Calder P.C., Pilling S., Baigrie R., Newsholme E.A. (1992) Plasma amino acid concentrations in the overtraining syndrome: Possible effects on the immune system. *Medicine and Science in Sports Exercise*, **24**(12): 1353–1358.

Paul A. A., Southgate D. A. T. (1978) *Mc Lance and Widdowson's The Composition of Foods*. HMSO: London, UK.

Phinney S. D., Bistrian B., Evans W. J., Gervino E., Blackburn G. L. (1983) The human metabolic response to chronic ketosis without caloric restriction: pre-servation of submaximal exercise capability with reduced carbohydrate oxida-tion. *Metabolism*, **32**: 769–776.

Pierson W. E., Covert D. S., Koenig J. Q., Namekata T., Kim Y. S. (1986) Implications of air pollution effects on athletic performance. *Medicine and Science in Sports and Exercise*, **18**(3): 322–327.

Péronnet F., Thibault G. (1989) Mathematical analysis of running performance and world running records. *Journal of Applied Pathology*, **67**(1): 453–465.

Peterkofsky B. (1991) Ascorbate requirement for hydroxylation and secretion of procollagen: relationship to inhibition of collagen synthesis in scurvy. *American Journal of Clinical Nutrition*, **54**: 1135S–1140S.

Pollock M. L. (1977a) Characteristics of elite distance runners: overview. *Ann. N.Y. Acad. Sci.*, **301**: 278–282.

Pollock M. L. (1977b) Submaximal and maximal working capacity of elite distance runners. Part I: cardiorespiratory aspects. *Ann. N.Y. Acad. Sci.*, **301**: 310–322.

Pollock M. L. (1973) Quantification of endurance training programmes. *Exercise and Sports Science Reviews*, **1**: 155–188.

Pollock M. L., Foster C., Knapp D., Rod J. L., Schmidt D. H. (1987) Effect of age and training on aerobic capacity and body composition of master athletes. *Journal of Applied Physiology*, **62**: 725–731.

Poole D. C., Richardson R. S. (1997) Determinants of oxygen uptake. *Sports Medicine*, **24**: 308–320.

Powers S. K., Dodd S., Freeman J., Ayers G. B., Samson H., McKnight T. (1989) Accuracy of pulse oximetry to estimate HbO_2 fraction of Hb during exercise. *Journal of Applied Physiology*, **67**: 300–304.

Powers S. K., Dodd S., Lawler J., Landry G., Kirtley M., McKnight T., Grinton S. (1988) Incidence of exercise-induced hypoxemia in elite athletes at sea level. *European Journal of Applied Physiology*, **58**: 289–302.

Powers S. K., Martin D., Dodd S. (1993) Exercise-induced hypoxaemia in elite endurance athletes. Incidence, causes and impact on $\dot{V}O_{2max}$. *Sports Medicine*, **16**: 14–22.

Pugh L. G. C. E. (1967) Athletes at altitude. *Journal of Physiology*, **192**: 619–646.

Pugh L. G., Corbett J. L., Johnson R. H. (1967) Rectal temperatures, weight losses, and sweat rates in marathon running. *Journal of Applied Physiology*, **23**, 347–352.

Qamer M. I., Read A. E. (1987) Effects of exercise on mesenteric blood flow in man. *Gut*, **28**: 583–587.

Ramsbottom R., Brewer J., Williams C. (1988). A progressive shuttle run test to estimate maximal oxygen uptake. *British Journal of Sports Medicine*, **22**: 141–144.

Ramsbottom R., Nute M. G. L., Williams C. (1987) Determinants of five kilometer running performance in active men and women. *British Journal of Sports Medicine*, **21**: 9–13.

Ramsbottom R., Williams C., Kerwin D. G., Nute M. L. G. (1992) Physiological and metabolic responses of men and women to a 5-km treadmill time trial. *Journal of Sports Sciences*, **10**: 119–129.

Rehrer N. J., Brouns F., Beckers E. J., ten Hoor F., Saris W. H. (1990) Gastric emptying with repeated drinking during running and bicycling. *International Journal of Sports Medicine*, **11**: 238–243.

Rennie D. W., Park Y., Veicsteinas A., Pendergast D. (1980) Metabolic and circulatory adaptations to cold water stress. In: Cerretelli P., Whipp B. J. (eds), *Exercise Bioenergetics and Gas Exchange*. Elseview/North Holland Biomedical Press: Amsterdam, The Netherlands, pp. 315–321.

Robergs R. A., Roberts S. O. (1997) *Exercise Physiology: Exercise Performance and Clinical Application*. Mosby: St Louis, USA, pp. 668–669.

Robertson R. J., Gilcher R., Metz K. F., Skrinar G. S., Allison T. G., Bahnson H. T., Abbott R. A., Becker R., Falkel J. E. (1982) Effect of induced erythrocythemia on hypoxia tolerance during physical exercise. *Journal of Applied Physiology*, **53**: 490–495.

Robblee N. M., Clandinin M. T. (1984) Effect of dietary fat level and polyunsaturated fatty acid content on the phospholipid composition of rat cardiac mitochondrial membranes and mitochodrial ATPase activity. *Journal of Nutrition*, **114**: 263–269.

Rowbottom D. G., Keast D., Morton A. R. (1998) Monitoring and preventing overreaching and overtraining in endurance athletes. In: Kreider R. B., Fry A. C., O'Toole M. L. (eds), *Overtraining in Sport*, Human Kinetics: Champaign, IL, USA, p. 47–66.

Sabatin P., Portero P., Gilles D., Bricout J., Guezennec C. Y. (1987) Metabolic and hormonal responses to lipid and carbohydrate diets during exercise in man. *Medicine and Science in Sports and Exercise*, **19**: 218–223.

Saltin B. (1990) Anaerobic capacity: Past, Present, and Prospective. In. Taylor A. W., Gollnick P. D. (eds) Biochemistry of Exercise VII Human Kinetics: Champaign, IL 387–412.

Saltin B. (1996) Exercise and the environment: focus on altitude. *Research Quarterly in Exercise and Sport*, **67**(3): 1–10.

Saltin B., Åstrand P.-O. (1967) Maximal oxygen uptake in athletes. *Journal of Applied Physiology*, **23**: 353–358.

Saltin B., Larsen H., Terrados N., Bangsbo J., Bak T., Kim C. K., Svedenhag J., Rolf C. J. (1995a) Aerobic exercise capacity at sea level and at altitude in Kenyan boys, junior and senior runners compared with Scandinavian runners. *Scandinavian Journal of Medicine and Science in Sports*, **5**: 209–221.

Saltin B., Kim C. K., Terrados N., Larsen H., Svedenhag J., Rolf C. J. (1995b) Morphology, enzyme activities and buffer capacity in leg muscles of Kenyan and Scandinavian runners. *Scandinavian Journal of Medicine and Science in Sports*, **5**: 222–230.

Sahlin K. (1992) Metabolic factors in fatigue. *Sports Medicine*, **12**(2): 99–107.

Sawka M. N., Pandolf L. B. (1998) Effect of body water loss on physiological function and exercise performance. In: Gisoli C. V., Lamb D. R. (eds), *Perspectives in Exercise Science and Sports Medicine, Vol. 3, Fluid homoeostasis during exercise*. Benchmark Press: Carmel, USA. pp. 1–25.

Schantz P. G., Henriksson, J. (1987) Enzyme levels of the NADH shuttle systems;

measurements in isolated muscle fibres from humans of differing physical activity. *Acta Physiologica Scandanavica*, **129**: 505–515.

Schmidt V., Bruck K. (1981) Effect of a pre-cooling maneuver on body temperature and exercise performance. *Journal of Applied Physiology*, **50**: 772–778.

Scott C. B., Roby F. B., Lohman T. G., Bunt J. C. (1991) The maximally accumulated oxygen deficit as an indicator of anaerobic capacity. *Medicine and Science in Sports and Exercise*, **23**: 618–624.

Scott B. K., Houmard J. A. (1994) Peak running velocity is highly related to distance running performance. *International Journal of Sports Medicine*, **15**: 504–507.

Scrimgeour A. G., Noakes T. D., Adams B., Myburg K. (1986) The influence of weekly training distance on fractional utilization of maximum aerobic capacity in marathon and ultramarathon runners. *European Journal of Applied Physiology*, **55**: 202–209.

Sen C. K. (1995) Oxidants and antioxidants in exercise. *Journal of Applied Physiology*, **79**: 675–686.

Senay L. C., Mitchell D., Wyndham C. H. (1976) Acclimatization in a hot, humid environment: Body fluid adjustments. *Journal of Applied Physiology*, **43**: 786–796.

Shepley B., MacDougall J. D., Cipriano N., Sutton J. R., Tarnopolsky M. A., Coates G. (1992) Physiological effects of tapering in highly trained athletes. *Journal of Applied Physiology*, **72**: 706–711.

Sherman W. M., Costill D. L. (1984) The marathon: dietary manipulation to optimize performance. *American Journal of Sports Medicine*, **12**(1): 44–51.

Sherman W. M., Costill D. L., Fink W. J., Miller J. M. (1981) Effect of exercise-diet manipulation on muscle glycogen and its subsequent utilization during performance. *International Journal of Sports Medicine*, **2**(2): 114–118.

Sherman W. M., Leenders N. (1995) Fat loading: the next magic bullet? *International Journal of Sports Nutrition*, **5**(Suppl.): S1–S12.

Sherman W. M., Plyley M. J., Sharp R. L., Van Handel P. J., McAllister R. M., Fink W. J., Costill D. L. (1982) Muscle glycogen storage and its relationship with water. *International Journal of Sports Medicine*, **3**: 22–24.

Simon-Schnass I. (1993) Vitamin E and high-altitude exercise. In: Packer L., Fuchs J. (eds), *Vitamin E in Health and Disease*. Marcel Dekker: Basel, Switzerland, pp. 455–463.

Simon-Schnass I., Pabst H. (1988) Influence of vitamin E on performance. *International Journal of Vitamin Nutrition Research*, **58**: 49–54.

Sjödin, B., Jacobs I. (1981) Onset of blood lactate accumulation and marathon running performance. *International Journal of Sports Medicine*, **2**: 23–26.

Sjödin B., Jacobs I., Svedenhag J. (1982) Changes in blood lactate accumulation (OBLA) and muscle enzymes after training at OBLA. *European Journal of Applied Physiology*, **49**: 45–57.

Sjödin B., Svedenhag J. (1985) Applied physiology of marathon running. *Sports Medicine*, **2**: 83–99.

Smith J. A. (1995) Exercise training and red blood cell turnover. *Sports Medicine*, **19**: 9–31.

Spencer M. R., Gastin P. B., Payne W. R. (1996) Energy system contribution during 400 to 1500 metres running. *New Studies in Athletics*, **11**(4): 59–65.

Spreit L. L., Gledhill N., Froese, A. B., Wilkes D. L. (1986) Effect of graded erythrocythemia and metabolic responses to exercise. *Journal of Applied Physiology*, **61**: 1942–1948.

Squires R. W., Buskirk E. R. (1982) Aerobic capacity during acute exposure to simulated altitude, 914 to 2,286 meters. *Medicine and Science in Sports and Exercise*, **14**: 36–40.

Staab J. S., Agnew J. W., Siconolfi S. F. (1992) Metabolic and performance responses to uphill and downhill running in distance runners. *Medicine and Science in Sports and Exercise*, **24**: 124–127.

Strydhom N. B., Kotze M. E., van der Walte W. H., Rogers G. G. (1976) Effect of ascorbic acid on rate of heat acclimation. *Journal of Applied Physiology*, **41**: 202–205.

Svedenhag J., Saltin B., Johansson C., Kaijser L. (1991) Aerobic and anaerobic exercise capacities of elite middle-distance runners after two weeks of training at moderate altitude. *Scandinavian Journal of Medicine and Science in Sports*, **1**: 205–214.

Svedenhag J., Sjödin B. (1984) Maximal and submaximal oxygen uptakes and blood lactate levels in elite male middle- and long-distance runners. *International Journal of Sports Medicine*, **5**: 255–261.

Svedenhag J., Sjödin B. (1985) Physiological characteristics of elite male runners in and off-season. *Canadian Journal of Applied Sport Sciences*, **10**: 127–133.

Svedenhag J., Sjödin B. (1994) Body-mass-modified running economy and step length in elite male middle- and long-distance runners. *International Journal of Sports Medicine*, **15**(6): 305–310.

Tabata I. (1996) Effects of moderate-intensity endurance and high-intensity intermittent training on anaerobic capacity and $\dot{V}O_{2max}$. *Medicine and Science in Sports and Exercise*, **28**: 1327–1330.

Tarnopolsky M. A. (1994) Caffeine and endurance performance. *Sports Medicine*, **18**(2): 109–125.

Tipton C. M., Mathes R. D., Maynard J. A., Carey, K. A. (1975) Influence of physical activity on ligaments and tendons. *Medicine and Science in Sports and Exercise*, **7**: 165–175.

Toner M. N., McArdle W. D. (1988) Physiological adjustments of man in the cold. In: Pandolf K. B., Sawka M. N., Gonzalez R. R. (eds), *Human Performance Physiology and Environmental Medicine at Terrestrial Extremes*. Benchmark Press: Indianapolis, USA, pp. 153–197.

Tremblay A., Boilard F., Breton M. F., Bessette H., Robergs A. F. (1984) The effect of a riboflavin supplementation on the nuritional status and performance of elite swimmers. *Nutritional Research*, **4**: 201–208.

Turner M. (1996) How 'biotech' drugs may win at Atlanta. *The Daily Telegraph*, 24th July p. 16.

Tsintzas K., Liu R., Williams C., Campbell I., Gaitanos G. (1993) The effect of carbohydrate ingestion on performance during a 30-km race. *International Journal of Sports Nutrition*, **3**: 127–139.

Van der Beek E. J. (1991) Vitamin supplementation and physical exercise performance. *Journal of Sports Science*, **9**(Special Issue): 77–89.

Van Erp-Bart A. M. J., Van Saris W. H. M., Binkhorst R. A., Vos J. A., Elvers J. W. H. (1989) Nationwide survey on nutritional habits in elite athletes, part II. Mineral and vitamin intake. *International Journal of Sports Medicine*, **10**: SS11–S16.

Van Zyl C. G., Lambert E. V., Hawley J. A., Noakes T. D., Dennis S. C. (1996) Effects of medium-chain triglyceride ingestion on fuel metabolism and cycling performance. *Journal of Applied Physiology*, **80**: 2217–2225.

Vukovich M. D., Costill D. L., Fink W. J. (1994) Carnitine supplementation: effect on muscle carnitine and glycogen content during exercise. *Medicine and Science in Sports Exercise*, **26**(9): 1122–1129.

Wagner P. D. (1996) Determinants of maximal oxygen transport and utilization. *Annual Reviews in Physiology*, **58**: 21–50.

Walker J. B. (1979) Creatine biosynthesis, regulation and function. *Adv. Enzymol*, **50**: 117–142.

Warhol M. J., Siegel A. J., Evans W. J., Silverman L. M. (1985) Skeletal muscle injury and repair in marathon runners after competition. *American Journal of Pathology*, **118**: 331–339.

Weiss S. J. (1989) Tissue destruction by neutrophils. *New England Journal of Medicine*, **320**: 365–376.

Wenger C. B. (1988) Human heat acclimatization. In: Pandolf K. B., Sawka M. N., Gonzalez R. R. (eds), *Human Performance Physiology and Environmental Medicine at Terrestrial Extremes*. Benchmark Press: Indianapolis, USA, pp. 153–197.

Wenger H. A., Bell G. J. (1986) The interaction of intensity, frequency and duration of exercise training in altering cardiorespiratory fitness. *Sports Medicine*, **3**: 346–354.

Weston A. R., Myburgh K. H., Lindsay F. H., Dennis S. C., Noakes T. D., Hawley J. A. (1997) Skeletal muscle buffering capacity and endurance performance after high-intensity interval training by well-trained cyclists. *European Journal of Applied Physiology*, **75**: 7–13.

Wilkinson D. M., Fallowfield J. L., Chapman L., Matthews A. (1997) The effect of a 7-day taper on simulated half-marathon performance. *Journal of Sports Sciences*, **15**: 135.

Wilkinson D. M., Fallowfield J. L., Myers S. D. (1999) A modified incremental shuttle run test for the determination of peak shuttle running speed and the prediction of maximal oxygen uptake. *Journal of Sports Sciences*, **17**(5) 413–419.

Williams C., Nute M. G., Broadbank L., Vinall S. (1990) Influence of fluid intake on endurance running performance. A comparison between water, glucose and fructose solutions. *European Journal of Applied Physiology*, **60**: 112–119.

Williams K. R. (1990) Relationship between distance running biomechanics and running economy. In: Cavanagh P. R. (ed.) *Biomechanics of Distance Running*. Human Kinetics: Champaign, IL, USA.

Williams K. R., Cavanagh P. R. (1983) A model for the calculation of mechanical power during distance running. *Journal of Biomechanics*, **16**: 115–128.

Williams K. R., Cavanagh P. (1987) Relationship between distance running mechanics, running economy, and performance. *Journal of Applied Physiology*, **63**: 1236–1246.

Wilmore J. H., Costill D. L. (1994) *Physiology of Sport and Exercise*. Human Kinetics: Champaign, IL, USA.

Witt E. H., Reznick A. Z., Viguie C. A. Starke-Reed P., Packer L. (1992) Exercise, oxidative damage and effects of antioxidant manipulation. *Journal of Nutrition*, **122**(Suppl. 3): 766–773.

Wolski L. A., McKenzie D. C., Wenger H. A. (1996) Altitude training for improvements in sea level performance: is there scientific evidence of benefit? *Sports Medicine*, **22**(4): 251–263.

Wood D. M. (1999) Assessment of maximal oxygen uptake in runners: new concepts on an old theme. Unpublished Doctoral thesis. University College Chichester, UK.

Wood D. M., Myers S. D., Fallowfield J. L. (1997) Non-linear $\dot{V}O_2$-running speed relationship in well-trained runners: implications for the assessment of running speed at VO_{2max}. *Proceedings of the Second Annual Congress of the European College of Sport Science, Copenhagen, Denmark*. pp. 944–945.

Woodhall A. A., Britton G., Jackson, M. J. (1997) Carotenoids and protection of phospholipids in solution or in liposomes against oxidation by peroxyl radicals: relationship between carotenoid structure and protective ability. *Biochemica et Biophysica Acta*, **1336**: 575–586.

Woodhall A. A., Lee S., Weesie R. J., Jackson M. J., Britton G. (1997) Oxidation of carotenoids by free radicals: relationship between structure and reactivity. *Biochemica et Biophysica Acta*, **1336**: 33–42.

Wyndham, C. H., Strydom N. B. (1969) The danger of inadequate water intake during marathon running. *South African Medical Journal*, **43**(29): 893–896.

Young M., Fricker P., Maughan R. (1998) The travelling athlete: issues relating to the Commonwealth Games, Malaysia 1998. *British Journal of Sports Medicine*, **32**: 77–81.

Index